NOTES

From a GAPS Practitioner

MW00462372

Notes From A GAPS Practioner ©2016 by Amy Mihaly. All rights reserved. This book is not intended as a substitute for the medical advice of a licensed practitioner. The reader should regularly consult with a practitioner in matters relating to his/her health and particularly with respect to any symptoms that may require diagnosis or medical attention.

No part of this book may be reproduced in any form or by any electronic or mechanical means including information storage and retrieval systems without permission in writing from the publisher, except by a reviewer who may quote brief passages in a review. Published by What If? Publishing, 133 E. 4th Street, Loveland, CO 80537, 970-667-0292. First Edition.

Any use of the letters GAPS in this publication are used solely as an acronym for *Gut and Psychology Syndrome*. *Gut & Psychology Syndrome* is the original work of Dr. Natasha Campbell-McBride and is her copyright. It is used in this book with her permission.

Cover and interior design: Liz Mrofka
Copyediting and proofing: Amy Mihaly
Printing: CreateSpace

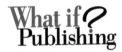

What If? Publishing
133 E. 4th Street
Loveland, CO 80537
WhatIfPublishing.com

ISBN-10: 0-9983300-1-9
ISBN-13: 978-0-9983300-1-3

NOTES

From a GAPS Practitioner

Using Diet to Unlock
the Body's Healing Secrets

Amy Mihaly

Acknowledgments

I would like to thank the many people who have supported me through the years. Without you I would not be who I am today.

This includes my family, my church family, and my friends who love and support me. Also my teachers, classmates, peers and patients who have encouraged me in my studies and made me dig deeper for real answers.

Thank you to my editors, Brian and Samantha; my publisher Liz, and my business coach Robin. I couldn't have done this without you.

And most of all, I would like to thank God, my Father, who has lovingly walked with me through every moment of my life, and who will be there for all that are to come. I am proof of His strength working through my weakness.

Table of Contents

Introduction

So here you are, reading this book. Maybe you have been doing GAPS for a while, but feel like you need a little more help and understanding. Maybe you are looking into GAPS to decide if it is something that you or your family should do. Maybe you are a grandparent, wondering about this crazy way of eating that your grandchild just started. Maybe you are health practitioner, looking for a way to better help your patients. No matter why you are reading this, this book is for you.

These reflections come not only from my practice as a GAPS practitioner, but as someone who has followed the GAPS protocol for over two years and experienced healing through these principles. This book is full of concepts, principles, and the word-pictures I have created to help understand the complexities of the human body and the incredible ability it has to heal itself when given the proper tools. The ideas contained in this book are ones I review regularly, and I turn to them when I don't understand right away what is going on in my body, or in the body of one of my patients. In reading this book, I hope that you will come away with a fundamental understanding of human nutrition to guide your decisions, as well as a helpful framework for understanding GAPS to improve your success in the process.

Note: The letters GAPS in this book are used solely an acronym for Gut and Psychology Syndrome™. Gut and Psychology Syndrome is the original work and copyright of Dr. Natasha Campbell-McBride, and is used with her permission.

Before You Read This Book:

As I sat down to write this book I tried to think of what I wished I understood before I started GAPS. These things are here. This book is written to be read first chronologically, then to be used as a reference over and over again. Please underline, dog-ear, and otherwise mark up this book—it is written to be a resource for you.

What This Book Is Not:

This book is not a comprehensive book about the GAPS diet. I do not discuss each stage of the Introduction diet, or every possible outcome and symptom you may experience, or the scientific details of metabolism and the like.

This book is meant to be a companion to the work of Dr. Natasha Campbell-McBride, including *Gut and Psychology Syndrome*, and other resources.

What This Book Is:

I wrote this book to give you an overall picture of what's going on in your body before, during, and after healing. It is also meant to be a guide to understand your body, and to highlight the things that are important and practical. My brain works by simplifying and categorizing the seemingly complex. Because our bodies are different, and because there are so many components at work, the mix of imbalances and injuries can have an infinite number of manifestations. This creates very different symptoms in each person, but the root problem is often simple. I have found that applying this simplification has been beneficial for others, as well as myself. My hope is that after reading this book you can begin to see through the smoke and mirrors of seemingly complex symptoms, into the true and often straightforward problem that needs addressed.

Find Support and Community

My goal for this book is for you to have it as a resource and reminder. There are different challenges with the GAPS protocol, but often the hardest thing is remembering why you are doing it and keeping back the fear. The fear because you think you may be crazy. You worry that you may be hurting your body, or that of your child's. You are surrounded by voices that have a very different view of disease and health. It can be easy to question yourself and why you thought you knew better. You do know better. You can know your body, and you should be the one making decisions about your body and your health. I want to give you resources to empower you, and help you remember. It may be through this book (and hopefully more to come), through my blog and the Be Well Clinic Community, through the *My Daily Insights: A GAPS Journal*, or a one-on-one appointment with you. I am on your team, and I want to empower you to take control of your health!

Fair warning: you will find it hard to unlearn the things you read in this book. This is a rabbit-hole of knowledge, and once you know, there is no turning back. If you don't want to commit to a long-term care of your health, stop reading this book! With knowledge comes responsibility, and that is not always easy to handle. But if you are sure that you want to come further down into the rabbit-hole, then keep reading!

—*Amy Mihaly*

Chapter One

Gut and Psychology Syndrome™

Gut and Psychology Syndrome, also know as GAPS, is referring to the link between the gut and the brain[1]. But what does that actually mean? Keep reading —we will explore what this syndrome is, and why we are seeing so many more disease of inflammation, allergies, mental illnesses, and more? Our children seem to be much sicker than ever, and in comparison, our parents and grandparents seem as "healthy as an ox." What changed? Is it our food? Immunizations? Better diagnosing? Crowded classrooms? Urban lifestyles? Toxin exposure? To answer that question, we first need to look at the body, and how it functions.

The Body

The body is made up of multiple organ systems that each have a specific job. The cardiovascular system pumps blood and brings oxygen, the digestive system absorbs our food, the muscular system helps us move, and so on. To perform even one of these "basic functions," dozens, hundreds, or thousands of pieces need to be perfectly in place. But when we are deficient in important nutrients, if we can't make proper hormone signals, or if we have clouded neurological pathways, those body functions begin to break down. The body is amazing, and can compensate, or work in a different way, for a long time, but eventually the problem will be seen. We know about these problems because of how our body reacts, what we call symptoms. Each symptom we experience tells us something about what is going on in our body, and by tracing these, we can often figure out how to correct the problem. When the problem is corrected, the symptom will disappear, because the body no longer needs to send you that distress signal. A healthy body is a quiet body!

All these wonderfully complex systems, which work together in a myriad of ways, don't work alone. The parts of us that are us (our own DNA), make up only about 10% of our body. Every system and function of our body works in conjunction with our symbiotic partners, or our flora, that make up the human microbiome.

The Human Microbiome

The human microbiome refers to the collection of bacteria, viruses, parasites, worms and other micro-organisms that live in our bodies. Scientists are now realizing that we are designed to work with these organisms in a partnering, symbiotic way. They believe that our bodies are made up of (up to) 90% of other creatures' DNA. We are really a shell, housing this wonderful partnership at work, which lets us function, live, and thrive.

Our microbe partners do things like help us with metabolism, detoxification, digestion of our food, protection from environmental toxins, communication with our immune system, and more. They talk to our hormones and are part of the hormone chain through which everything functions. They also help us maintain our enterocytes, which make up the lining of the gut wall. These cells are designed to be the barrier of the intestines—allowing only digested food into the bloodstream. (If you would like to learn more about this, NPR put out a great animated video about the human microbiome on YouTube. It is only a few minutes long, and I recommend watching it. Just search NPR and human microbiome).

These days, most people have heard of gut flora. But we have flora everywhere, not just in our guts! Members of this microbiome are found in our lungs, throat, mouth, and ears; on our scalp and skin, in our armpits, in and around our organs, everywhere! The mix of flora depends on the location, moisture, pH, and purpose of that area. But all that other flora comes from your gut! The intestines are the breeding ground of the flora that populates your body. Because they are linked, if something causes your gut flora to be unhealthy, the flora around your entire body becomes unhealthy as well.

All microbes produce different types of substances—some are helpful, and others are harmful. Can you guess which kind of substances unhealthy flora produces? That's right, toxic ones! And those harmful substances love to leak into our bodies and cause damage.

Our microbiomes are fascinating, and much more time could be exploring their intricacies. The important thing to know is that the flora in our bodies perform many important tasks, and without them we cannot survive. It's also important to know that we cannot live in a microbe void—if we do not have good microbes partnering with our bodies, bad ones will take over. So we need to create and maintain an environment that encourages friendly and helpful microbes to live in our body. We will explore this further in the next chapter[4].

GAPS (aka Leaky Gut Syndrome)

As we have already said, the acronym GAPS stands for Gut and Psychology Syndrome, but it also stands for Gut and Physiology Syndrome. In real words, it stands for "problem in the gut will lead to brain (mental) disease," and "problem in the gut will lead to body (physical) disease." It is confirming what physicians have known, starting with Hippocrates, that *all diseases begin in the gut*. It may sound like a simplified and primitive view of disease, but let's explore how this may be true.

According to Dr. Campbell-McBride, GAPS manifests itself in a myriad of symptoms, potentially affecting every body system, in multiple possible ways. Some of the common symptoms of GAPS syndrome are anxiety, depression, asthma, food allergies, autoimmune disease, OCD, schizophrenia, memory loss, arthritis, fatigue, muscle wasting, dyslexia, ADD/ADHD, autism, diarrhea, constipation, ulcers, heart disease, high cholesterol, the list goes on.

When you look at the list above, these symptoms don't seem to have any connection with each other. Additionally, many of these things are already bundled into sets of symptoms we call "diseases." How can joint pain and dyslexia be caused by the same thing? How can those possibly be related?

To answer this question, we need to trace these symptoms back to their roots. A symptom is what you experience when your body is trying to tell you something? For example, it may be letting you know that it is being attacked, or that it is not able to function properly because it is missing something. So, if a symptom is being experienced, we need to figure out why the body is sending that signal. We need to figure out what is wrong, what is at the root[1].

Damage to the Flora

A leaky gut begins with damage to the gut lining. Let's look at a common scenario showing the breakdown of a healthy gut. First, something damages the gut flora. This may occur from antibiotics, steroids, birth control, anti-depressants, ibuprofen, antacids, or many other medications. The flora could also be damaged from an exposure to metal, toxins or chlorine in the water, vaccine administration, or a serious illness. If the flora is not strong enough to recover, or if the damage is ongoing, the cells lining the intestines, called enterocytes, begin to suffer. Among the many roles that the gut flora performs, one important job is that of maintaining the health of these enterocyte cells. In a healthy body, enterocytes create a tight wall of cells lining the intestines and any substance, before it can enter the bloodstream, is analyzed and processed inside one of these cells. But without the upkeep of the gut flora, the enterocytes will become old, worn-out, sickly and unable to absorb food. They also become unable to maintain their tight junctions. This leads to substances such as undigested food particles and toxins entering the bloodstream uninhibited.

Next Comes Malnutrition

Gut flora plays a vital role in making sure our bodies have the nutrition they need. In a healthy person, the flora lining the gut helps with the digestion of our food. When we eat a vegetable filled with vitamins and minerals, it is our gut flora that helps us get that nutrition off of the fibrous stalk and into our bodies. Different species of gut flora produce enzymes to help us break down our food, and others produce vitamin and minerals themselves. Healthy gut flora is in constant communication with our body, and—depending on the present metabolic needs of the body—different flora can produce some of the different nutrients that are needed. These substances are made on-demand in the intestines, then absorbed quickly into the bloodstream to be used by the body in whatever way needed.

When we lose these helpful microbe partners, our body can't get the nutrients it needs to perform at full capacity. Cells can't replicate as often, damaged cells can't be repaired, and metabolic pathways won't be able to function properly because they are missing vital ingredients or activators. The body may not be able to produce enough of a hormone such as serotonin; epigenetics (gene expression) may become altered; and hungry organ systems —such as the brain and immune system—will have to function at an impaired level. All cells, including the enterocytes lining the intestines, will be affected.

A Leaky Gut is Born

So a leaky gut is actually that! Physical holes develop between the sick enterocytes, allowing undigested food particles, toxins, and other unwanted substances into the bloodstream. The level of toxicity in the body quickly increases, and allergies start developing to the different food protein particles that have entered the bloodstream before being fully broken down. These processes can lead to further problems, such as anaphylactic reactions and autoimmune disease. Additionally, the lack of gut flora, and the compromised enterocytes lead to different nutritional deficiencies, and the body is not able to maintain optimal functioning or heal damaged areas of the body.

Toxins

What is a toxin? There are many definitions of toxins, but I prefer this one: A toxin is something in the body that is not helpful to the body. I'll say it again—*a toxin is a substance in the body that is not helpful to the body*. Toxins could be chemicals or pesticides, highly processed (changed) food particles, proteins that our body has developed an allergy to, heavy metals, substances produced by unhealthy gut flora, pseudo-estrogens, excessive histamine in the body, free radicals, and more. It is anything that does not help the body, but rather creates more work for the body. Toxins are not good.

Toxins are harmful to us, and difficult to deal with. And the more that are present, the more our detoxification systems will have to work. When the primary detox organs (liver and lungs) get overwhelmed and overloaded, the body will rely more heavily on other ways to deal with the toxins, such as sending it out through the skin, or storing it in fat cells. When these are no longer enough, toxicity symptoms will be frequent, and often constant. These symptoms can include fatigue, brain fog, headaches, tinnitus, seizures, eczema, mood disorders, anxiety, and many more! When the body is unable to contain and control the toxins, they are allowed free range of the body, which spells disaster for you and me!

Most toxins have an affinity to a certain type of tissue or organ type. Their

Case Study: A Look at Dyslexia

Dyslexia occurs when the brain does not correctly receive or process the signals it is receiving from the ocular nerve. What causes this broken analysis? Scientists have now found a link between certain toxins and some disorders, like dyslexia[3]. But where did the toxins come from? As we have just learned, they come either from environmental exposure or unhealthy gut flora. When we see a symptom like learning difficulties, we understand that there is probably a breakdown of the barrier in our gut lining. Through this breakdown, toxins enter the bloodstream and spread throughout the body. Some of these toxins have an affinity for brain tissue, and their presence causes neurotransmitter imbalance, damaged brain cells, and incorrect sensory interpretation. In certain situations, this causes the symptom we know as dyslexia.

Some of you scholars may remember that our brains have an extra defense in place, one that should provide protection to our brain from these invading toxins. And you are right! The blood-brain barrier is designed to provide special protection to this vital organ. But much like the defenses on the outside of our body can fail, the blood-brain barrier can be breached as well. Malnutrition, combined with repeated toxin assault on the blood-brain barrier, leaves the brain vulnerable to toxins. And when there are many toxins present in the brain, it is difficult to process through the noise and veil of the toxin soup, and things like dyslexia, dyspraxia, and other learning disabilities will appear.

affinity will determine where they do damage. Toxins are also attracted to areas of weakness, like an overworked joint or a strained organ. Because of the illness, injury or fatigue in that area, toxins are able to enter in, cause damage, and even settle down to live there. This is a problem, because long-term toxin presence can even cause further complications like parasite overgrowth, organ failure, and perhaps even cancers.

Inflammation Sets In

When a leaky gut is present, inflammation in the body quickly increases. Inflammation is a non-specific response to a threat to the body, and it is regulated by the inflammatory arm of the immune system. Inflammation is triggered by toxin damage, reaction to proteins (allergies), or physical injury (broken arm), among other things. This is a normal and healthy response of the body, and inflammation plays a large role in keeping the body clean and repaired. However, when there is repeated damage from a constant flow of toxins and undigested food particles, this arm of the immune system becomes overwhelmed.

Case Study: Causes of Joint Pain

Let's trace joint pain back to the root cause. What causes joint pain? It's inflammation, right? Just like when you sprained your ankle in high school basketball (OK, that was me!), you experienced swelling, redness, pain, and heat. Because inflammation is a non-specific immune response that is initiated anytime something goes wrong in the body. Following that logic, then joint pain is caused by something being wrong in the joint. But what caused the injury? If you did not take a long hike, or get hit on the football field, or fall off your bike, how did damage occur? The most common reason for this damage is something we have already talked about—toxin damage. Certain toxins with affinity for cartilage cause damage in the joint. The body initiates the inflammatory response: rushing fluid, heat, redness, pain—the whole nine yards. When the toxins are cleaned up, the pain and inflammation goes away, and you probably will forget that the joint ever hurt. But if there are too many toxins, or if the immune system is not functioning properly, then the toxins cannot get cleaned out of the joint, and the pain and inflammation will continue. In time, chronic joint pain, arthritis, or even the autoimmune disease rheumatoid arthritis may develop.

Calling in Reinforcements

As this arm of the immune system become overwhelmed, it calls on the other arm of the immune system to help. This second arm, or humoral immunity, is our specific immune response. It contains things like our memory T cells, which remember diseases and attack any stray invaders before a full infection can reoccur. The ability of our immune system to mark and remember disease, and protect our body is amazing, but when it becomes overactive, it can lead to serious problems. This excessive activity comes when the inflammatory arm of the immune system is overwhelmed, and the humoral arm steps in to help out. The arms of the immune system get out of balance, leading to things like anaphylactic reactions and autoimmune disease. This process is more complicated then what I just described, and I recommend Dr. Campbell-McBride's work for further details.

But when we seal up the gut lining again, the flow of offending substances and toxins will stop. The damage from these will decrease, and with it, inflammation. When inflammation begins to get back under control, it allows the activity of the humoral arm of the immune system to decrease, and any specific attacks of protein or tissues will calm down. Over time the tissue will heal, memory T cells will be shelved, and inflammation will happen at a proper and manageable rate. All from healing and sealing up the gut lining!

Immune System Command

In addition to the two arms of the immune system, the other part of the immune system we need to talk about is the command center. This command center of the immune system is located around the intestines, making up about 80% of our immune system. This is often referred to as GALT (gut associated lymphoid tissue). Constant communication occurs between the gut flora inside the intestines, and our immune system sitting right outside it. When we eat something that contains harmful bacteria, like salmonella for example, our flora informs our immune system, which then mounts an attack in response. In another function, when we eat a food, like peanuts, it is our gut flora that tells our immune system that this is, in fact, a food, and that it does not need to be attacked. When there is breakdown in this communication system then issues like chronic illness, allergies, and many other problems may result. Of course, the communication between the immune system and the gut flora is more numerous and complex than what I have just described, but you get the idea[1].

Looking at the Root Problem

So, in review, when we trace symptoms like dyslexia and joint pain back to the root, what do we find? We find one common root—the gut! The cells of the intestines have been allowed to become unhealthy; the gut flora is lacking in helpful microbes while being overpopulated with harmful ones; and the rest of the body has become overrun with unhealthy microbes and damaging toxins. The problems compound from there. The body's detoxification system become overwhelmed and broken, hormones get out of balance, and our immune system begins attacking erratically and incorrectly. Immune symptoms build, toxin damage increases, and malnutrition shows itself in deficiency disease and weight problems. Sounds pretty awful and hopeless, right?

But this is good news! How can I say that? This is why we walked through the exercise of tracing to the root of the symptoms. Because how do we relieve symptoms? *By correcting the problem.* What is the root problem? *A body that has too little good gut flora, too much bad gut flora, and unhealthy barrier cells.* **To correct all the symptoms that occur from this root problem, we simply need to heal and seal the gut lining, and restore a healthy microbiome.**

And this is the focus of the GAPS protocol. It is designed specifically to provide the necessary nutritional building blocks to repair and rebuild the enterocytes that make up the protective barrier of the gut, and to supply and feed good microbes, so the balance of the gut can be restored. We are going to look at the GAPS protocol in more detail in the next chapter.

Chapter Two

Now that we know how we got here, let's talk about how we can fix it. The body is always wanting to healing itself—we just need to provide it with what it needs to repair and clean itself up. And the GAPS protocol is about just that.

What is the GAPS Protocol?

The GAPS protocol is a nutritional healing protocol designed to heal a leaky gut, or gut dysbiosis. For most people, it is temporary and only needs to be strictly followed for a period of time.

It was designed by Dr. Natasha Campbell-McBride, MD more than fifteen years ago. Motivated by her belief that nutrition was key to healing, she returned to school to get a Masters degree in nutrition. Using her knowledge of the human body and how it works, and ideas from other healing diets, she created the GAPS nutritional healing protocol. Many natural practitioners agree that her protocol is the most efficient way to heal a leaky gut. If followed for the recommended time (this varies, but is often around 1.5-3 years), many see tremendous improvement, if not cessation, of the symptoms that are occurring.

Is GAPS for You?

Like anything else, there is no guarantee that this is what your body needs. Let me say that again. I am not promising you that GAPS is the answer to all your health problems! The body is complicated, and there are many factors that play into health problems. It is important to research your symptoms, and make sure they are linked to inflammation and a leaky gut and not something else, like cancer. It is best to work with a certified GAPS practitioner, or at least another practitioner that is familiar and open to nutritional healing, so they can help you on this journey. That being said, the vast majority of symptoms are from "diseases of inflammation," which you will soon see is linked directly to a leaky gut. And if your current health conditions are a result from a leaky gut, there is a good chance that following this healing protocol will benefit you.

But let's answer the question a different way. What is GAPS? The GAPS diet is returning to a traditional way of eating, with an emphasis on certain foods that are incredibly nourishing and healing to your body. It is eating real and good-for-you foods. We all need to eat food, and we all know we should eat healthy food. So, on one hand, the GAPS diet is eating as we have eaten for thousands of years (with the exception of the last 60-100 years). This is very similar to the Weston A. Price diet. This diet has been dubbed the "well-person diet," whereas the GAPS diet is the "healing," or "sick-person diet." As I said before, the unique quality of the GAPS diet is the emphasis on healing foods.

Defining the Protocol

GAPS is not just a diet, it is a healing protocol. There are three aspects to the GAPS healing protocol: diet, detoxification, and supplementation. All of these aspects are important, and without observing all of them, your chances of success are limited.

PART ONE: THE DIET

We will talk about this more in later chapters. In summary, there are three phases to the GAPS diet; the Introduction Diet, the Full GAPS Diet, and the Coming off GAPS Diet (or transitioning to the well-person diet).

Introduction Diet

The Introduction, or Intro Diet, is a progression of six stages. These stages begin with nutrient dense, easy-to-digest foods, and, as healing occurs, foods that are more difficult to digest are added. The focus of these stages is gut soothing, healing, rebuilding and microbial repopulation. The Intro Diet is often done in the beginning of a person's GAPS journey, but it can be re-done at any time, like if old problems resurface, or during an illness. This is true especially of stages 1-3, which I believe is the most powerful and efficient rebuilding protocol there is. Again, this book is not about the exact stages, so they are not discussed in detail here.

Full GAPS Diet

On the Full GAPS diet you can eat a large variety of foods, with the exception of processed sugars, simple carbs, and starches. Most of your time in GAPS is usually spent here. It is very important to continue with the main healing foods at this stage. This is not merely about "legal" and "illegal" foods. The ratio of foods matter! Meat stock, animal fat, and probiotic foods need to be consumed daily, and in large amounts, if you want healing to continue. Fruits, nuts, and other "goodies" need to be limited. It is easy to want to rush this stage, or grow lax in eating the right foods, as many days you may feel pretty good. Resist the temptation to move forward too quickly! It takes time to establish the changes in your body, and Full GAPS is the time to do this!

During this period you may also experience a health rollercoaster. You may have some good days, or weeks, then experience a setback, or an increase or return of symptoms. This is very discouraging, but don't quit! This is a normal part of the healing process, and if you continue (sometimes minor adjustments are needed), you will get back on track, and often ahead of where you were before the setback. At any time during Full GAPS, you may choose to go back through the Intro Diet to provide a "healing boost"—perhaps to accelerate healing or to help your body through an exposure or illness.

Coming Off the GAPS Diet

Six months to a year after your symptoms have resolved (especially gut symptoms), you can begin the final phase of the diet—Coming Off the GAPS diet. You slowly begin adding foods like small potatoes, beans, sourdough bread, and buckwheat, millet and quinoa. At this point, if your body is tolerating these types of foods, it would likely be helpful to look into the Weston A. Price diet, as that traditional way of eating, or "well-person diet", is beneficial to follow for the rest of your life. Enjoy the freedom of eating whatever real food your body can handle! Processed foods should be consumed rarely, if ever. It was from eating these fake foods that much of the damage occurred in your body in the first place. If you return them to a significant part of your diet again, you will likely end up in the same place as before. And when your body is functioning as it should, if you do occasionally eat them, your body will process any toxins present in them, and they should do no lasting harm to you.

PART TWO: DETOXING

Detoxing is important for several reasons. First, we are exposed to large amounts of toxins through what we put on our skin and the air we breathe. Second, toxins are being produced inside our bodies as well. Most bad, or pathogenic microbes are producing toxins that leak directly into our bloodstream in large amounts. Third, GAPS often leads to damaged detoxification systems. This damage may have been from a large, one-time toxin exposure, malnutrition that caused organ fatigue or failure, or just from being overwhelmed by the slow and steady inflow of toxins over time. In any case, we need to help our detoxification system in its job of cleansing the body until it is functioning well enough to take back over. How do we do this? First we start with what I refer to as "gentle detoxing."

Sunbathing

Daily time outside in the sunlight is a form of detoxification. Direct exposure of our skin to the sun allows the body to detox, and is a great way to clean our bodies. Begin with 5-10 minutes in the sun, working your way up to 1-2 hours or more. As you regularly do this, and increase your fat intake, you will find that you do not burn very easily, even if you are fair-skinned! Do not put sunscreens on your skin, as this adds more toxins to your skin and blocks the detox pathways and the body's ability to make vitamin D from the sunlight. If you need to be in the sun longer than your skin can handle, it is best to cover up with clothing and a hat, and you may use coconut oil or other natural products that have small amounts of SPF.

Detox Baths

Detox baths are another important part of this protocol and are beneficial in detoxification. Let's start with water! It is best to dechlorinate the water for your detox baths, as chlorine is a harmful chemical, and it kills everything it comes into contact with, including the good microbes on your skin. If you do not have a whole-house filter, you can use a carbon shower filter or a bath dechlorination ball (my favorites are listed on bewellclinic.net/Resources). You can take a full bath, or just a foot bath. The pores on the bottoms of your feet are large, and the body can easily eliminate toxins through your feet. To the dechlorinated water you should add ½-1 cup of one of the following agents: baking soda, raw apple cider vinegar, or Epsom salts. It is good to rotate these, and you may find that you can tell which one your body needs that day. You should stay in the water for at least 20 min, although you can stay longer, and the temperature should be warm to hot. The temperature of the water does matter, and if it is too hot it will cause you to detox more quickly.

I like to think about the goal of detox bathing this way: it is to clean out the toxins that are currently circulating in the bloodstream, but avoid initiating cellular detox. If the water is too hot, or you stay in too long, or you put too much of the detox agent in, you will start to experience unpleasant symptoms like headache, brain fog, nausea, or racing heart. These symptoms show an increase in blood toxins, probably because the cells are starting to dump their toxins into the bloodstream. It is best to get out of the bath immediately if you start experiencing these symptoms. Drink water, lie down for a while, and it usually passes quickly. Make a note for the next time, and simply decrease the heat, amount of detox agent, or amount of time to avoid the same experience. Again, your goal for this activity should be a gentle, enjoyable detox, after which you feel lighter and more energized. If you feel heavy, irritable, tired or nauseated (similar to feeling sun-sick, or after a massage), you probably caused more toxin release than your body was able to handle. This happens to everyone, don't worry. As with everything in this journey, just observe what you did and how it made you feel, and note it for later (more on this in chapter 7). However, there is no need to take a cold bath, as this can increase your stress response and work against healing.

Oil Pulling

Oil pulling is a simple method of detoxification. It involves holding about a teaspoon of organic olive oil or coconut oil in your mouth for 20-30 minutes once or twice a day. Swish the oil between your teeth (stay to the front of your mouth, no need to gargle). This pulls the toxins out of your gums, teeth and skin, depositing them in the oil. At the end of your time, spit the oil in a trash can (oils can clog your drains) and brush your teeth with the remainder of the oil in your mouth. The oil also softens the plaque on your teeth, making it easier to remove. For a little extra whitening, you can dip your toothbrush in baking soda before brushing.

If you have a strong gag reflex, try distracting yourself with a movie or a book until you get used to the activity. If the oil suddenly tastes awful, spit it out! Especially in the beginning, your mouth may dump a large amount of toxins into the oil, and the taste will change, signaling you to get it out! Even if it hasn't been 20 minutes, you can brush your teeth and be done for the day—detoxing still happened. You may notice that your teeth change colors when you begin oil pulling—these are the toxins leaving your teeth, and when they are clean your teeth will be white again! The best time to oil pull is in the morning, on an empty stomach, but you can do it anytime—find something that works well with your schedule!

Juicing

The last major detoxification support recommended is juicing. We will talk about juicing in detail in the future chapter on cleansing, but I will briefly say this: juicing is one of the oldest and gentlest methods of detoxification, and once the body is tolerating fresh vegetables (Intro, Stage 4), it is an important part of your daily routine. If you believe your symptoms stem largely from a toxin overload or exposure, it is especially important to juice once or twice a day.

PART THREE: SUPPLEMENTATION

The final part of the GAPS protocol is supplementation. It's preferable to get all the nutrition we need from the food we eat, but that's not always possible. Much of the food we can buy or grow today has fewer nutrients in them today because our soil itself is depleted of nutrients. Also, many people who suffer from GAPS lack the gut flora, enzymes, or healthy enterocytes to extract the nutrition that is available in a food. Finally, particular nutrients may be severely depleted in someone's body, and it would take a very long time to replenish those nutrients through food alone. For these reasons, certain food-based supplements are recommended for those following the GAPS protocol. Most people should take fermented cod liver oil with high vitamin butter oil, omega-3 fish oil, probiotic capsules, and use iodine on their skin. Many people also find that desiccated liver capsules are an easier way to get their daily dose of liver. Certain people will need specific vitamin or mineral supplementation, but this is generally decided on a case-by-case basis, and should be discussed with your GAPS practitioner.

Remember, the reason for supplementation is largely to replenish deficient nutrients and to assist the body as it heals. When healing has occurred, you may find that you no longer need certain supplements, as your body may be able to get what it needs from the nutrient-dense foods you choose to eat.

The GAPS Protocol in Real Life

I know what you're thinking. I still haven't told you what this protocol really means for you. As you read this book, my hope is that you will get a better picture of what it may look like for you. But I also want to tell you in plain English, what GAPS means.

GAPS Is . . .

1. It is realizing that the root cause of most symptoms (inflammatory, immune, toxic, or hormonal) is a fundamental imbalance in the environment of the body. When you change the environment of your body, you should expect to see changes in your symptoms and reactions.

2. It is accepting that your decisions about things like food, sleep, skin care products have an effect on your health. You get to be in charge of how you feel. GAPS means taking responsibility.

3. It is regularly choosing certain foods over others because those foods are helpful to what your body needs right now. While there are guidelines about what to eat and not eat, you need to practice listening to your body, It can tell you what it needs that day.

4. It is a temporary protocol. You are going to be eating those foods for a period of time (1.5-3 years for most) to allow healing and (hopefully) lasting change. It means voluntarily following a strict protocol long enough to make and establish the desired changes, in order to gain the enormous benefit of healing and freedom after completing it.

5. It is a lifestyle change. GAPS is not about replacing your normal recipes with the same, but GAPS approved ones. It is about thinking differently about what you eat, and knowing why you eat it. It is about restoring food to its proper role of nourishment and satisfaction, not relegating it to entertainment and coping. When you are done with the GAPS protocol, and have more freedom to eat other foods, you will know what foods to choose, because you know the affect it will have on your body.

6. It will probably be one of the hardest things you ever do. But the rewards and payback on the other side are just as profound. You can do it! And there are ways to make it easier (such as working closely with a Certified GAPS Practitioner, and being part of a GAPS community and/or having another strong support system).
   Ultimately, you are the one who puts the work in, and only you get to fully experience the rewards of that work!

7. It means making a lot of decisions. No good decision is ever wasted! No matter how imperfectly you do the protocol, or how many times you cheat and restart, or even if you just implement one part, like daily meat stock, you are supporting a better body environment.

8. It is a learning experience. Few people are very in tune with their bodies, but you can be. Be patient with yourself. Accept the role of student, not expert. Approach with the intention to observe and learn, and you will be more successful overall, no matter how many "setbacks" you experience. The only way to fail is to quit forever. Keep getting back up.

9. It may not be the right thing for you right now. Occasionally the GAPS protocol is not the best option for healing at a certain point in time. You can read more about this in chapter 9. Most people do benefit on this protocol, but there is no magic bullet to fix anything, and that is also true of this protocol.

What's the Difference?

The difference between the GAPS protocol and other diets like Paleo, AIP, FODMAPs, or even the SCD diet, is that it's not just about legal and illegal foods. GAPS emphasizes eating lots of nutrient dense foods instead of merely staying within some guidelines. For example, you can follow a grain-free diet, but still eat a diet consisting primarily of nuts and fruit. While these foods are allowed even on the GAPS diet, they are not nutrient dense foods with high amounts of specific compounds that healing the gut lining. In fact, they may still feed bad flora, like candida, that may be causing many of your symptoms. The difference between GAPS and other diets is the emphasis on eating certain healing foods in large amounts, and other, less helpful foods in small amounts. It's about changing the environment, which we will talk about in more detail later.

What If I Have Already Tried . . . And Failed . . . GAPS?

Some of you are probably reading this book as a last resort, because you know you need to do GAPS, but can't seem to stay with it. You are trying to find anything that will help you. Here is what I have to say to you. Yes, there are good and helpful things in this book, and that is the reason for writing this book, but there may be something else in your way. It's not physical, but it can be one of the hardest things to overcome: guilt and insecurities about past failures on GAPS or other diets. Let me say something very clearly here. You have not failed! Every good choice you have made for your body has made a positive difference in your body. Restarting GAPS, or partially doing GAPS, or stopping any good habit you started but couldn't continue, is not failure!

This so-called "failing" GAPS happens all the time. Don't be discouraged; it takes many people multiple tries before they can stay on the GAPS protocol for the desired length of time! Take each "failure" as a learning experience, prepare a little more (mentally and physically) for the next time and, when the time is right, start again. Each time you restart the GAPS diet you'll be more successful, because you are closer to understanding what your body is feeling, and what it's asking for. This is especially true if you are coming from a fast-food background—there is a lot to learn! Even people who regularly cooked before GAPS can find it time consuming and difficult to keep up with the demands in the kitchen, especially if you are cooking for more than yourself. Often we "fail" from lack of knowledge or preparation, not from lack of desire or willpower. Every time you learn something new, you increase your chance of success the next time!

And even if you can never seem to do GAPS "right", you still have not failed. Every day you eat good, healing nutritious foods, you are doing good for your body. So if you do GAPS for a week, you have done good to your body in that week. It's not time lost. As I said before, GAPS is most efficient when you follow the protocol exactly. But the principles of healing still apply, no matter your pace. So don't stay in discouragement (it's normal to feel something—it's hard when our expectations are disappointed). But when you're ready, get up and keep going forward! It's not failing, it's learning! And pretty soon, you are going to be quite a learned person!

Chapter Three

In this chapter, I would like to introduce the metaphor I use to think about the body, and the changes that have to happen inside, as healing occurs. Like all metaphors, this one is not perfect, but it gives you a good picture about what is happening in your body, and why it takes so long. At the end of the chapter I also wrote down the metaphor I use when explaining this to children. Tempting as it is, don't skip over that part! Simple is often the most helpful, and when you are doing something as challenging and complicated as the GAPS protocol, you need something that is easy to hang onto.

The Environment Metaphor

Picture, if you will, your body—the inside of your body. Think about all the functions it performs, and the many workers in every cell, helping that cell perform its task. Got it? Okay, now picture your body as a neighborhood. There are workers and residents, systems that produce and gather, or clean up, and infrastructure supporting it all.

Now, think about the different types of neighborhoods there are. There are downtown, vintage neighborhoods, suburban neighborhoods with HOAs and soccer moms. There are ritzy neighborhoods, celebrity neighborhoods, apartment neighborhoods, run-down neighborhoods, and country acreages.

Now let's contrast two very different types of neighborhoods. I know I am using stereotypes here—it is the clearest way to show differences. My goal is not to cause offense, but to create a simple and relatable metaphor to different health states of the human body.

Think about the difference between an upscale neighborhood, such as a gated community, and an impoverished area of a big city. Very different communities, right? But what is it exactly that makes them different? Is it the people? Access to resources? Street lights? Sanitation services? The presence of bus stops? What is it that makes a neighborhood what it is?

A Tale of Two Neighborhoods

Let's look at the gated community first. There are beautiful manicured lawns, an HOA that regulates everything from trash on your property, weeds and grass length, and maybe even cars parked in front of your house. Each house is painted a different color than the house next door, and there is no visible peeling paint or broken gutters. There are street-lights everywhere. Everything is clean and open. People are well-behaved, and smile back at you. There's not a lot of noise, especially after 10pm.

Next, let's look at the impoverished area, what people may call "the slums." What does that community look like? It's dirty, with trash everywhere.

People have old-looking, and sometimes broken-down cars parked on the street. There's at least one bus stop, which is crowded much of the day. At night a homeless man sleeps on the bench. The only grass is down the street at the empty lot, but it is four feet high, mostly covered with garbage and an unwanted couch. On the entire street, there are only two streetlights—and one of them is out. There is no enforced noise ordinance; in fact, the fights usually start around 10pm. People don't go outside much, because it's not safe—there's rampant crime and drug use. It's rare to see a smile.

They are very different, right? And there isn't just one thing that makes it different—there are many factors that contribute to the environment of a particular neighborhood. However, the structure and infrastructure has a large effect on attracting, or allowing people from certain socio-economic statuses to live in this or that community.

Your Body is a Neighborhood

Our bodies are an environment as well, a neighborhood environment. And, for most of us, they're somewhere between the two communities. Chronic disease, malnutrition, poor eating, or bad lifestyle habits will create an environment that looks a lot like "the slums." Our insides are not very clean—there's a lot of toxicity—we get headaches and are tired all the time, we are depressed or anxious, and it takes precious energy to work, be productive, and even to smile sometimes. But wouldn't we all like to resemble a gated community? A picture of health with radiant skin, full of life and hope. Productivity at work, and energy left over to pursue hobbies.

So How Do We Get From One Neighborhood to the Other?

Many people suggest changing your body's environment by taking probiotics. Bring in the right neighbors, and the neighborhood will improve. But is that how it works? Can we just send in good people? What if we sent the most popular humanitarian workers, or priests, or even just a really good family into our "slums"? Would that work? No! Why not? Because the environment hasn't changed. It's still unsafe. It's still dirty. Those people—if they stay—are going to be fearful like everyone else in the neighborhood. There are going to be problems. They may move out the first chance they get, they may be killed, or they may just become exhausted from not sleeping well at night.

The same thing would happen if we do the opposite in the gated community. What if a drug dealer, or meth-addicted family moved into the gated community? Are they going to last very long? No, they're not. Why? Because their neighbors will be uncomfortable. They will call the cops the first time any rule is broken. They will put a lot of pressure on them to move away. Those people aren't going to stay in that environment any more than the other family will stay in the slums.

In the same way, the "residents" in our bodies—our flora, or microbiome, are going to be determined based on the physical environment.

If we have a clean and organized body (like the gated community), we're going to attract good, helpful microorganisms. If we have a run-down, toxin-filled environment, then we're going to attract unhealthy and unhelpful microorganisms.

We want to clean up our bodies, so we attract the right kind of "neighbors."

Making the Change

How do we clean up? We need to bring in dumpsters and clean up the trash, install streetlights, and tear some buildings down. We need to rebuild or update apartments, and turn the empty lot into a park. Before long, our slums will transform into a budding urban community. And as these changes happen, more and more of the "right" kind of people will move in. At some point the balance will shift, and we can say that the neighborhood has changed.

Change of any kind takes time and a lot of work. It can't happen overnight, and unless resources continue pouring into the area for a period of time, it will soon go back to the way it was. But with persistent energy and the right building blocks, the old "slums" area could be the next real estate hot spot.

It is no different in your body. As you are doing work with the GAPS protocol, you are doing just this. You are eating foods that heal your leaky gut. You are cleaning up the toxic trash that's in your body, and by doing so, you are inviting (not to mention swallowing) the neighbors you want to take up residence in your gut. This is why it takes time to see real healing, and even more time to maintain it. When the focus is true rebuilding—not just a quick facelift—it should take a while.

The Kids' Environment Metaphor (aka the Fairy-Tale Land Metaphor)

Children (and adults) do really well with this metaphor—even at a pretty young age. It helps them understand and accept the difficulties that go along with doing the GAPS protocol. I mention this here briefly, so parents can go through this exercise with their kids, but I have found that it can be helpful for adults as well.

First, think about a villain in fairy tale. Now think about where they live, and what it looks like.

If they are having problems thinking of something, you could suggest something like the overgrown castle in Sleeping Beauty.

What does it look like?

It's overrun with weeds. There are thorns and ravens everywhere. It's dark, scary, and not a good place to be, right?

That's our bad neighborhood. That's what your body kinda looks like right now.

Now think about some beautiful place—the place from a fairy tale that you wish most you could visit. What is it?

Maybe Pocahontas' new world? Or the beautiful castle of Cinderella?

What is it that you love about it? Why do you like it? Do you want your body to be like that?

You don't want an overgrown castle with thorns and a dragon, do you? Don't you want to have this beautiful, clean, and light place? So how do we get there?

You get there by choosing, every day, to do the little, right things, and not the wrong things.

The right things are detoxing (helping your body clean out); eating the right foods; and making the right choices in sleeping, what you put on your skin, and more. All those little choices that you make every day are important, and they will improve your body's environment.

Each day you get to decide whether you want to drink your stock today. Or eat a bite of sauerkraut. Or eat a cookie. All those choice have an outcome, and the outcomes will build up over time.

These choices, over time, will change the environment of your body. But the good news is, you get to choose what you want your body to look like—which environment you want to create.

Even young children are surprisingly capable and interested in making good decisions when they understand the consequences.

Do You Want The Good Guys Or Bad Guys To Win?

This is a question I ask all the children I talk to about GAPS. But I also ask it of myself, and I encourage you to ask yourself this question as well, especially when it's a struggle to make the right choice.

Just remember, if you eat that cookie (etc), you're helping the bad guys win. When I think of that, something rises up from deep inside me, a desire to help good triumph over evil! And that often gives me enough resolve to make the better choice. Remember, right now, you are fighting a battle. And you get to help the good guys win by giving them food, and rest, and by cleaning out the trash. And each time you choose something good, the bad guys are that much closer to losing. So take up the battle cry, and march onward!

What Kind of Shape Is Your Neighborhood In?

Now that we have discussed neighborhoods in general, think about the "neighborhood" in your body. How does it look? Take a few minutes to create an honest picture of where your body is at. Your neighborhood is probably not a Chicago slums, but it's probably not Beverly Hills either. Think through your neighborhood. What shape are the buildings in? How much trash is littering the streets, or hiding in dark corners? Is there life, light, and energy present like a thriving downtown? Or is it a sleepy retirement community? Do you have a picture? Great!

Now think about what you want your neighborhood to look like? Is there less trash, more life, stronger structures? What kind of people live there? Are they thriving and productive? You get to build this neighborhood, and you get to decide what is important and what it should be like. Keep picturing it until you have built a picture you love! Solidify that picture in your mind. I would encourage you to find a way to remember this picture—write or draw it out, or print out a photo that reminds you of your ideal neighborhood. This is what you are working toward, and when things get hard, this picture will help!

It may also be helpful to have a picture of where you were when you started —a picture of your run-down neighborhood. When you feel like you have been working hard but have seen no changes, a quick look at your original neighborhood will likely reveal how far you have actually come! Once you get these pictures (no, really! Stop reading this book and get these pictures—we'll wait for you) we will talk about how we are going to make the changes that we need. The next few chapters are about the three major components needed for your neighborhood renewal—the Building Blocks, the Cleaners, and the Residents.

Chapter Four

Building Blocks

As we discussed in the Environment Metaphor, in order to make positive changes in the body we need to do a lot of work—building up, cleaning up, and moving in new neighbors. Let's focus on the building blocks first. Building blocks are substances that our body needs to build a strong and healthy structure. And contrary to what we have been told all our lives, most foods that densely provide these are from animals, not from plants.

Keep Reading To Find Out Why

As Dr. Campbell-McBride describes in her online article, "Feeding versus Cleansing," animal foods primarily rebuild our bodies, while plant foods primarily cleanse. This is the reason why a long-term vegan diet is so harmful to the human body: regardless of how careful we are to eat clean, normal breakdown of cells will occur. Our bodies were not designed to recycle 100% of the essential fatty acids and proteins that are released during the breakdown of cells when they die; rather, we were designed to rebuild cells from a constant new supply from the foods we eat. These are found in animal foods, where the structure is very similar to our bodies (since we are in the animal kingdom[1]).

When there has been damage from toxins—or when there is malabsorption and malnutrition present—the need for these nutrient dense animal foods is even higher. I have found that, after starting the GAPS diet, children and adults go through a short period of time where they cannot seem to get enough to eat. They may eat a full meal every 1.5-2 hours. This is normal and expected, and usually lasts about a month, although it may last longer. After that, most people seem to eat large portion sizes for the next six months to a year, then their intake of food decreases. It is very important to eat as much as the body wants you to eat! When you are eating good, nutrient-dense foods (not empty calories, as most of us are used to eating), you will not gain unwanted weight or feel ill, even if you eat as much as you want. However, if you restrict your intake, you are limiting your body's ability to rebuild and repair, causing your healing to occur more slowly.

What are Nutrient-Dense Foods?

Nutrient-dense food is weighed by the following requirements: the quantity of vitamins, minerals, amino acids, proteins, animal fats, and essential fatty acids that are present; how much of these are actually available to be absorbed by the body (bio-available); and the ease with which the body can digest and absorb them. Nutrient-dense foods can be whole, partial (extracted), raw, or cooked in various ways. Let's look at exactly what that means.

Quantity of Nutrients

Not all foods are created equal. Different types of food have different nutrients in them, and differing amounts of those nutrients. For example a carrot contains moderate levels of Vitamin C and low levels of zinc[5]. Liver, on the other hand, contains high amounts of Folate but low amounts of Vitamin C[4]. Each food is unique. The nutrient levels listed by the USDA for each food are an average, and the true nutrient levels of, for example, the carrot that you are eating will vary depending on how that food was grown. Some factors that help determine the nutrients available in a food are: the nutrients available in the soil or feed during growth, the season and global location of growth, and the amount of access to sunlight. When looking for nutrient-dense foods, the density (amount) of nutrients present in a food is the first thing to look at.

Bio-Available Nutrients

The bio-availability of nutrients does not refer to the amount of nutrition that is in the food, but to how many nutrients are accessible to the body. If one food has more total Vitamin A, but only 15% of it is absorbed; and a second food has less Vitamin A, but 95% of it is absorbed by the body, then the second food has more bio-available nutrients in it.

This contrast can be seen between plant and animal products. Vegetables have lots of vitamins and minerals in them, but many of those are so tightly bound up in the fibers of the vegetables, it is difficult for our body to absorb a large amount of them. For our body to be able to use these vitamins, we need many different enzymes, and healthy gut flora, to break off and absorb the nutrients that are present. Meat has more bio-available nutrients. Not only do animal products contain good amounts of vitamins and minerals, these nutrients are much easier for our body to digest and absorb. Therefore, animal products are often more nutrient-dense than plants. The nutrient density of a food is also determined by the amount of nutrients that are available for the body to use.

Preparation Matters

We can make food easier to digest and absorb by changing the way it is prepared, therefore making it more nutrient-dense. Different methods of preparation are appropriate for different categories of food. Plants (fruits, vegetables and grains) are better digested when fermented or cooked, and when eaten with plenty of fat. Animal products are usually easier to digest raw, or boiled in water (meat stock). Preparing food differently can make it more nutrient-dense because the nutrients that are present made to be more available[8].

Pair with Fat-Soluble Activators

Finally, to increase the body's ability to get nutrients, it is important to pair your food with animal fat. Animal fat contains fat-soluble activators. Your body needs these substances to absorb and use many of the different nutrients from plants and animals. When these activators are missing or are few in number, the body may not be able to use even bio-available nutrients. Additionally, eating fat with a meal slows the absorption of sugar, so the blood sugar is less likely to spike after eating. It is important to control the increase of blood sugar, because a drastic increase can lead to all sorts of unpleasant symptoms. High blood sugar can also change the way the body uses and stores nutrients and energy reserves. Eating fat with any food makes it more nutrients dense because you are supplying the body with the fat-soluble activators it needs[7].

Aren't Raw Veggies Better?

Now, you may be wondering about the enzymes present in fresh fruits and veggies. I just said that we need enzymes to extract vitamins, and then I told you to kill them by cooking them. Yes, that is true. This is a case of doing what is best for the body at this time. Enzymes do help us break down these foods, but with GAPS, the few enzymes and beneficial microbes that are present are not able to help much. Without the additional help from your body, the enzymes that are naturally present in the raw food are probably not enough to do the job. This is why it's best to avoid eating raw fruits and vegetables in the beginning stages of healing. Until the body is up for the challenge of vitamin extraction, several methods can be used to make the nutrients easier to absorb. We can use heat, microbes, or manual extraction (juicing) to begin the breakdown process, and we can pair them with foods containing fat-soluble activators to increase absorption and assimilation (use) of nutrients.

Breakdown by Heat

When we cook plants, we break down the fibers that are present in them. Cooking a fruit or vegetable until it is soft begins to free the nutrients held inside, making it easier for the body to remove and absorb them. And if you boil those vegetables in a stock, you make it even easier to access the nutrients, because many of them are now suspended in the stock or soup you are drinking, ready to be absorbed by the body[8].

Breakdown by Fermentation

We can also get more nutrition out of our plants by fermenting them. Fermentation of vegetables is the process of adding beneficial bacteria to something (usually a vegetable) in a closed environment, so they combine. The bacteria go to work on the vegetable, breaking down the cell walls, extracting nutrients, creating enzymes, and multiplying their helpful little selves. The result is a wholly helpful food—full of available vitamins and minerals, enzymes, and more.

Breakdown by Juicing

We can manually extract some of the vitamins in plants through the process known as juicing. The juice produced using this method is still primarily a cleansing food (more on this in the next chapter), but the nutrition available to our bodies is higher than if you ate those foods whole. Also, because much of the fiber is removed, you can consume a higher volume of these foods without unpleasant intestinal side effects, thus increasing your potential intake of nutrients by sheer volume alone.

Looking for a Better Nutrient-Dense Food

It takes a lot of work for our bodies to get nutrients from plants! This is why every culture throughout human history (with the exception of the modern vegan movement) consumes some type of animal product. Through the years, as people groups around the world have been studied, not one culture has been found that survived exclusively on plant matter. The form of animal food may not be what we consider meat—seafood, fat, insects, blood, eggs, milk, you get the picture. But in every instance, some form of animal product is consumed. This is because animal products are a nutrient-dense food, containing building blocks that the body can use to grow and repair itself. The body maintains a constantly balance of catabolic (breaking down) and anabolic (building up) activity. Because of our body's catabolic action, we need certain nutrients to rebuild. The cellular structure of animals is similar to our own, and animal foods provide the most efficient building blocks for our body's rebuilding. Not all animal foods are created equal, either. Certain foods from an animal like fat, organ meats, milk and eggs are more nutrient-dense then the muscle meats of an animal. It is important to eat these foods to support the body's repair and healing.

Meat Stock

Meat is most easily digested raw. Except for a few select dishes, most of us do not regularly consume meat in a raw form. Thankfully, we can still get benefit from meat in a cooked form. When you cook meat in water, creating a stock, you make it even easier to digest, and building blocks like collagen and essential fatty acids are pulled into the liquid stock, drastically reducing the amount of effort the body has to put forth before it can use it.

Now let me clarify. I am talking about meat stock, not bone broth. Bone broth, which has recently become very popular, is a great thing to consume. High amounts of amino acids and minerals are available in bone broth, but that includes something called glutamic acid. This is in the family of MSG, and for many people with GAPS, it can trigger symptoms they are prone to, including learning difficulties, headaches, migraines, and seizures. For that reason, meat stock (or short-cooked broth), is recommended when you begin GAPS. There are many resources talking about how to prepare the meat stock recommended on GAPS, so I won't describe it in detail here, but you should know that meat stock has a short cooking time (2-6 hours), and is primarily meat (80%), with some bones and joints (20%). It should be consumed daily, preferably at every meal. A general rule is this: the more meat stock you drink, the faster your gut lining will heal[2].

How to Drink More Meat Stock

It can be difficult to consume this amount of meat stock, so here are some different ways you can get this nourishing food in your body.

- In the morning, fill a thermos with heated stock so you can conveniently drink warm stock from it throughout the day.
- Poach your morning eggs in stock instead of water—then drink the stock along with your breakfast.
- Drink stock as your beverage with meals. This is especially helpful if you have a hard time feeling full. The stock seems to fill in those empty places in your stomach, especially when there is extra fat melted in.
- Eat your stock chilled, with a spoon. This is especially nice in the summer when it is more difficult to drink hot stock.
- Use your stock to make soups; don't just drink it plain all the time. You will enjoy the variety, yet still get in your daily stock.
- Drink stock between meals as a snack. Drop in an egg yolk or two to make it extra delicious and sustaining.

- If you are getting bored with the flavor, try adding different vegetables and herbs to your stock to change the taste.
- Don't forget to eat the meat from the stock as well as the liquid. Because of the shorter cooking time, the meat retains much of its flavor and nutrition.

Getting the Body's Building Blocks from Stock

Although we get many things from meat stock, one of the main building blocks we are looking for is collagen. Collagen is a protein structure that breaks down into gelatin, which is an amino acid present in our connective tissues throughout the body. There are many types of collagen, but the five most common are found in large amounts in our skin, tendons, ligaments, organs, bones, cartilage, eye, artery walls, capillaries, hair, cell surfaces, and more.

Other important substances we get from stock and broth are bone, marrow, molecules called proteoglycans, and amino acids like proline, glycine, glutamine, and alanine. All of these nutrients are necessary building blocks for essential structures in our body, such as cartilage, blood, intestines, immune system and more. Remember, these are already present in a usable form in the connective tissue, fat, muscle tissue, joints, fascia, and bones of the animal products. It is the method of cooking that makes them all so readily available for our body's use[8].

Muscle Meat Versus Meat

One confusion that arises in nutrition is from the definition of meat. When most people think of meat, they are thinking of muscle meat—chicken breasts, legs of lamb, rib eye steaks, and pork chops. But a more correct definition of meat would include any part of the animal, including organ meats, fat, skin, and connective tissue. These "extra" parts of the animal contain significantly higher amounts of nutrients then the muscle meats do. When only muscle meats are eaten, some problems can arise. They are high in protein, which can lead to constipation and Vitamin A deficiency if they are not consumed with enough fat. They have only low levels of some vitamins and minerals, which can lead to deficiencies if you are relying on meat to supply those nutrients. And many muscle meats are trimmed of fat, and have very little connective tissue, which are both large suppliers of the building blocks we just discussed.

When you eat other parts of the animal, not just the muscle meats, you will get more nutrients, balance your protein intake with fat, and eat plenty of the building blocks needed to repair and support the body. It can take some people a while to get used to the idea of eating things like chicken skin, joint cartilage and organ meats. If that is the case, I suggest blending these wonderful foods with your stock liquid in a blender. With a good blending, the texture of these food should no longer be a problem, and your body will have ready and easy access to the nutrients and building blocks in these foods. Eating this "extra" meat is essential to healing, and is a must while following the GAPS protocol. Whenever I refer to meat, I am using the broader definition, which includes more than muscle meat. If I mean just muscle meat, I will refer to it as such[2].

Other Preparations of Meat

Meat does not always have to be in the form of stock. Other methods of preparation are acceptable during the GAPS protocol, although different stages of the Introduction diet allow only certain types of meat preparation. This is because different preparations of meat are easier to digest than others. Boiled meat is easier to digest then baked or broiled meat, which is easier to digest than fried meat, which is easier to digest than grilled meat. Therefore, as you experience healing, your gut can digest and absorb nutrients from other preparations of meat.

Organ Meats

Organ meats—such as liver, heart, brain, and kidneys—contain concentrated amounts of nutrients. Liver is the most commonly consumed organ meat, and it is recommended to eat it regularly, especially while on the GAPS protocol. Many nutrients are found to be more concentrated in liver than anywhere else. Liver contains vitamin A, the B vitamins (especially B12), folic acid, iron (in a usable form), copper, zinc, chromium, CoQ10, purines, good quality protein, and an unidentified anti-fatigue factor[8]. This reason alone should cause all of us to eat liver on a regular basis. But we don't. Let's look at a few reasons why we don't, and how those reasons can be overcome.

Aren't Toxins Stored in the Liver?

Some people worry about liver being full of toxins. It seems only logical that the organ that processes toxins would, of course, be full of toxins. But let's investigate. Yes, the liver does process toxins, but toxins are not stored in the liver. They are actually stored primarily in fat cells. Only a very sick animal will have a liver full of toxins. So unless the liver looks sickly (believe me, you can tell), it can be assumed that it is largely free of toxins. That being said, it is best to avoid supermarket pork and chicken livers, unless they are pastured or organic, because these are likely to be from sick or sun-deprived animals, and probably have lower nutrient amounts.

What About Vitamin A Toxicity?

On the opposite side of the spectrum, others are concerned about developing Vitamin A toxicity from the high amounts that are present in the liver. This is true, it is possible to get too much Vitamin A from liver, but a person would have to consume very large amounts of liver on a consistent basis to develop problems. The few people who have developed symptoms, such as vomiting and drowsiness, from excessive Vitamin A had consumed an estimated several million units of Vitamin A in one sitting. Toxicity is not likely to occur even with regular consumption of liver. For an adult, it is recommended to eat two servings of 100-grams of liver per week, which contains about 50,000 IU of vitamin A per serving. Many people consume more than this, however, and studies show no ill effects even if you were to consume a full serving of 50,000 IU every day[7].

I Can't Stand The Taste, Texture or Smell

Many people know that liver is good for them, but they feel like they can't eat it for one of these reasons. Liver traditionally has a strong taste and smell, and the texture can be dry, crumbling, and overall unpleasant. But don't give up hope! There are many ways to regularly eat liver. You may find success in overcoming your aversion by trying some of the tricks listed below.

- Soak your liver in an acid, like lemon or whey, before cooking. This removes some of the unpleasant bitterness.
- Make liver and onions, with lots of fat! This is a traditional way to prepare liver, and for a few people, it brings back pleasant childhood memories (although not for everyone!)
- Boil the liver in your meat stock, and if it doesn't make it too strong (beef livers can be very strong), crumble or blend the liver into the liquid. This way of "hiding" the liver works very well.
- Make liver pate. This combines liver with fat and spices, making a rich and delicious spread (that can be eaten by the spoonful) that tastes only a little of liver.
- Make liver jerky. Cut your raw liver into strips and dehydrate it. The dehydration process seems to take some of the strong taste out of it. It also changes the texture.
- Freeze raw liver and grate it into foods. A little liver added to meatloaf or soup will not likely be noticed.

- Make or buy desiccated liver capsules. If you can get your liver no other way, or convenience and availability dictate, you can take your liver in a capsule form. There are several companies that produce good-quality products, and these can be found at bewellclinic.net/Resources.

Meat Needs Fat Too!

All meats, including organ meats, need to be eaten with a good amount of healthy animal fat. Vitamins A and D, and fat-soluble activators like K2, help the body get all the nutrition possible from the meat. Let's look at an example. When protein is absorbed, the body needs vitamin A to be present in order to use it. There is some vitamin A stored in the liver, but if that is not being regularly replenished by eating animal fats, the body will quickly become deficient. Because vitamin A is needed in order to utilize proteins, some activities within the body may begin to suffer from this functional lack of proteins (proteins are present, but without vitamin A, the body cannot use them). And this is only one example of the need of nutrients to pair with fat in order to be used.

Enzymes Also Help Digest Meat

Vegetables are not the only things that need enzymes in order to be digested —meat does too! Many people with GAPS are lacking the enzymes needed to digest meat or other animal products. This is why it is important to eat fermented foods with your meals. The beneficial microbes and the enzymes they produce, combined with any natural enzymes or enzyme stimulators already in your body, will aid in the digestion of the animal product. What you eat is important, but unless you can digest it, it does not have any benefit to you.

Fat is Essential to Life

Fat contains some very important building materials. However, the type of fat we should eat is another area of nutritional debate and confusion. To understand the importance of fat, especially saturated fat, in our body, we need to understand what parts of our bodies are made up of fat. Here are just a few examples detailing the role fat plays in our bodies.

Every cell membrane in our bodies is made up of at least 50% fat (with an even higher concentration in brain and nervous tissue). Our immune system needs fat to work well, and it is used to make many of our hormones—including androgens, testosterone, estrogen, progesterone, cortisol, and serotonin. Saturated fat is a major component in the intestinal wall. Our heart tissue prefers to use fat for energy, and the body uses cholesterol to repair any inflammatory damage that happens in our body. We make bile salts (used to digest fat) from fat, and we need cholesterol to make vitamin D. Fat plays an important role in our detoxification pathways. And the list goes on[8].

What About Cholesterol?

Now, with the mention of cholesterol, you may be wondering about all the dangers of high cholesterol. This discussion is (you guessed it) outside the purpose of this book. In short it is inflammation, not cholesterol, that is really linked to heart disease. Good, unbiased science has always proven this to be true, and recent studies have confirmed that eating animal fat does not have a negative effect on your health[3]. (If you would like to read more about this, I would recommend reading *Put Your Heart in Your Mouth* by Dr. Campbell-McBride.)

Nutrients Contained in Fats

All animal fats contain similar nutrients, although the exact ratio and amount of different molecules varies. To get an idea of what is contained in animal fats, let's look at the composition of butter. Butter contains the fat-soluble vitamins A, D, K1, and E, as well as their complement factors. They also contain other important nutrients like the Wulzen factor and Activator X (or vitamin K2). Different types of short and medium chain fatty acids are present, some of which are only found in a few foods. Butter and other animal fats contain arachidonic acid (AA), which plays a vital role in immune function. Omega-6 and omega-3 essential fatty acids are present in balanced ratios, and there are trace minerals including selenium, iodine, zinc, chromium, and manganese. Other nutrients in butter are conjugated linoleic acid, lecithin, cholesterol, and glycosphingolipids[6]. Each and every one of these nutrients provides amazing support to the body in one way or another.

Eat Your Fat

Bottom line: fat contains important building blocks, ones that we need for our neighborhood renovation project. So we need to eat fat, and we need to eat a lot of it! For most people, I recommend that they start by eating a ½ cup of added animal fat a day, and work up to 1 ½ cups of added animal fat a day. Now, unless you already make a habit of eating fat daily, even a half cup may make you feel full and nauseated. Start slowly, and work your way up. Remember how we need cholesterol to make bile salts, which digest our fat? If you are fat deficient, your bile production may not be operating at maximum capacity, and it may need some attention before it can catch up. Many people do fine by simply slowly increasing the amount of fat they eat, but others may need to take a bile supplement for a period of time. (Have you gotten a GAPS practitioner yet?) Fermented vegetables and apple cider vinegar also stimulate your digestive enzymes, and should be paired with fat consumption.

As with meat stock, the more fat you eat, the more quickly your body will heal. The brain, nervous system, hormones, immune system, gut lining, and joints are most helped by fat intake. You want to give your body as much of this as it asks for. Remember that I said to try eating 1½ cups of added animal fat a day? I said that for two reasons.

First, it helps to break any barriers against fat. Your body may ask you to eat that much fat (or more) on a daily basis, especially for a period of time. Like with everything else, you need to listen to what your body is asking for. By pushing to eat 1 ½ cups of fat a day, most people find that they have broken through any mental or physical barriers that would cause them to limit their fat intake. When they are fine with eating that much fat, if their body asks for 2 or 3 cups on a certain day, they will have no problem obliging.

Second, it provides an opportunity to notice how you feel when consuming that much fat. Many symptoms are greatly reduced just by increasing your fat intake. If you experience relief of your symptoms (such as joint pain, moodiness, memory or energy problems, stress intolerance, or frequent illnesses), then you need to keep eating fat! We all need to eat fat, but some need to eat more than others. Find out what works well for you. My goal, as always, is to help you be an expert detective; to listen to your body and work with it to provide what it is asking for.

Oil (Fat) Supplementation

Dr. Campbell-McBride recommends that all GAPS patients supplement their diet with three different types of concentrated, nutrient-dense foods: fish oil, cod liver oil, and nut and seed oils. If you would like more details then we discuss here, I would recommend the chapters in her book on fats and cod liver oil (*Gut and Psychology Syndrome*) as well as the Weston A. Price Foundation website. When supplementing essential fatty acids, caution should be used, especially if the person is prone to seizures or tics. Even if you don't have these symptoms, it is not uncommon to see some kind of reaction in people with severe fatty acid deficiencies when you begin a supplement. In these cases, supplementation is important, but caution should be used, so start with a small dose and increase gradually. If you experience symptoms, or suspect that you are very deficient in essential fatty acids, it is very important that you work with a practitioner familiar with this type of supplementation.

Fish Oil

When we think about oil supplements, fish oil may come to mind. Fish oil is rich in Omega 3, from which EPA (Eicosapentaenoic Acid) and DHA (Docosahexaenoic Acid) are formed. These two essential fatty acids are very important in brain and eye development and function. For people who have suffered from GAPS are deficient in the nutrients needed to convert omega 3 into EPA and DHA, it is important to consume a food or supplement in which that conversion has already been made. Cold-water fish and algae are rich in these essential fatty acids. The ratio of these essential fatty acids is also important, with a ratio favoring more EPA than DHA.

Cod Liver Oil

You may be surprised to learn that there is a difference between fish oil and cod liver oil. For most people with GAPS, both supplements are necessary to combat the body's long-standing nutritional deficiencies. In addition to providing EPA and DHA, cod liver oil provides vitamins A and D in a safe and helpful ratio. The vitamin A found in cod liver oil is already in the correct form to be used by the body, and cod liver oil is also the richest source of Vitamin D. I recommend only a few manufacturers of cod liver oil, as most cod liver oil is processed incorrectly and synthetic vitamins have been added, often in incorrect ratios. The ratios found in nature will be the best and safest for us to consume. You can find those recommendations on the Weston A. Price Foundation website, and the few that I have experience with are listed at bewellclinic.net/Resources. It is best to take cod liver oil along with something containing K2. Among other foods, this is found in butter. Dr. Price, who researched and used fermented cod liver oil extensively, found that high vitamin butter oil (high in vitamin K2) significantly increased the effectiveness of cod liver oil when taken together. As long as ghee or butter is tolerated, I recommend this combination for supplementation as well.

Nut and Seed Oils

Some of the essential fatty acids we need are found most densely in plants. These are mostly Omega-6 fats (or Linoleic Acid), which can form GLA (Gamma-Linolenic Acid), DGLA (Dihomogamma-Linolenic Acid), and AA (Arachidonic Acid). These have many important functions in the body, including the brain. Because the conversion to these essential fatty acids from Omega-6 requires additional nutrients, it is best to consume them in a form that already contains GLA, DGLA, and AA. The most important of these essential fatty acids is AA, which is a vital part of brain fat, and is used by the immune system. When it is severely deficient, it can cause the brain to shrink (visible on an MRI). The best sources of these (in descending order) are borage oils, blackcurrant seed oil, evening primrose oil, and hemp oil. Just like fish oils, many plant oils are not processed safely. It is important to check the manufacturing process. Plant oils, like all oils, should be stored in a cool, dark place. Heat, oxygen, and light all damage the oils and cause them to turn rancid and toxic.

Quality Matters

It is important to note that the quality of fat matters. For animal fat, pasture-raised is important, because exposure to the sun, and sun-exposed grass, is what produces many of the nutrients that should be present. Fat from animals that live in a barn all the time is going to have lower nutritional content than fat from pastured animals. Also animals, just like us, store toxins in their fat. For this reason it is best to purchase animal fat that is hormone and antibiotic free, at least. Plant fats need to be organic, truly cold-pressed, stored correctly, and not mixed (or cut) with any other oils. This information is often not disclosed on the packaging, so do your research. If these choices are truly not options in your budget, don't give up! Fat is more nutrient-dense, and therefore a better option, then pizza or doughnuts, no matter what the quality. And because of its protective and detoxifying properties, eating fat, even lower quality fat, will still work to protect your body from harm.

The quality of fat doesn't just have to do with how the animal or plant was raised, but also how the fat was processed. Many commercial lards and tallows, for example, use high heat and pressure—both of which destroy nutrients and create toxins. Fats processed this way can easily go rancid. There are a few commercial brands that have recently emerged which seem to sell a safe product, but my recommendation is to render your own fat whenever possible. Then you know what quality fat was used, how it was processed, and how old it is. Sourcing fat can be challenging, but you can search online, or contact the nearest Weston A. Price chapter for information about butchers near you. The actual rendering process is very simple, and only requires a little patience and time.

Hints to Eating More Fat

Unless you grew up doing it, eating this much fat can feel like a full-time job. Aside from the mental block, other hindrances can get in the way of eating all the fat our body needs. Here are a few suggestions for how you can eat more fat.

- Add fat to everything—every bowl of soup, every chicken breast, every vegetable!
- Eat fat on its own. I love to cube butter and eat it alone, or with fruit for a movie snack. I am also known to eat an entire tub of sour cream on the way home from the store (sometimes I even have a spoon).
- Plan your dishes around fat. Certain dishes automatically contain more fat than others. Choose these as often as possible.
- Eat egg yolks. Because of their high cholesterol content, egg yolks are considered fats. These can be eaten added to stock, as part of a GAPS milkshake, or in Russian custard.
- Don't get stuck in a rut. Butter is not the only fat! Try different fats—duck and goose fat, chicken fat, lard, tallow, and sour cream (creme fraische) are also great choices. Different fats are better paired with different dishes, and variety always helps!
- Use fat instead of water to cook meat, eggs or vegetables. If you need some extra lubrication to keep the food from burning or sticking to dish, use fat instead of water.
- When you are done cooking, pour the extra fat on top of your food, and eat it!
- Lick your plate! Not recommended during a dinner party, but for normal dining, consider . . . you paid a lot for that fat—don't waste it!
- Add fat to cooked fruit. Butter is best for this, but you can get away with a mild lard if you add some spices like cinnamon and nutmeg.

How to Eat Fat While Dairy Free

Eating enough fat can be challenging if you are dairy free (I know from experience). Most people find that a spoonful of lard or tallow is not very palatable on its own, but you can try adding it to each mug and bowl of stock and soup you eat. Fry your food as much as possible, and eat all the frying fat with the food. And don't forget about egg yolks—Russian custard is dairy free (you can find it in *Gut and Psychology Syndrome*). Also, see if you can tolerate ghee—many dairy-free people can. If you are not able to tolerate it now, you may be able to when some more healing has taken place.

Other Building Blocks

Our bodies are complex, and there are many more things needed than those listed in this chapter. Eating a varied diet, consisting of different vegetables and meats, will help ensure that you are giving your body access to what it needs. However, although we need windows and light bulbs to have a functioning house, a neighborhood is primarily made up of brick and mortar. Meat stock and fats are like trucks, full of these basic building materials, delivering to our front door. Bring in lots of these materials every day!

Chapter Five

Calling in the Cleaners

Let's talk about cleaning up! Earlier, when you imagined your current neighborhood, you probably saw dirt, trash, and dysfunction. Your neighborhood needs to be rebuilt, but much of it needs to be cleaned up first. So, who do you call? The cleaners!

First, let's talk about the normal ways your body cleans up. One of the most amazing functions in our body is its ability to process, remove, or store the toxins we are exposed to. At this point in history, we are exposed to many more toxins than our ancestors, but they did not live in a toxin-free environment. Smoke-filled houses, snake and insect bites, and exposure to lead and copper are only a few examples of the toxins their bodies encountered. The human body is designed to handle these exposures, and to prevent the toxins from causing permanent harm. We cannot avoid all toxin exposure, but we can support the natural body systems that are in place. We are going to discuss the three major players that protect our body from toxin damage. The first is a nutrient-rich diet, especially high in fats and fat-soluble nutrients. The second is inflammation, which is controlled by immune system. The third is our organs along the body's detoxification pathways.

Nutrient-Rich Diet

We discussed this at length in the previous chapter. Let me again emphasize here that a nutrient-rich diet protects us from damage from toxins. Healthy, functioning cells make up healthy, functioning organs. These healthy cells and organs repel damage, repair quickly, and regenerate easily. These activities are fueled by certain nutrients, and when those nutrients are present, any damage that does occur is quickly removed and healed. This is why the GAPS protocol so strongly emphasizes a nutrient-rich diet. Not only does it provide the building blocks of repair, it also strengthens the cells so they can do much of their own clean-up work. For someone who is very ill, the primary focus needs to be on diet, not cleansing, because healthy cells and strong structure are needed to safely clean and heal the body.

How Inflammation Promotes Healing

Wait! Inflammation is good? Yes, the reaction of inflammation, initiated by the immune system, is what the body uses to clean up damage in the body. We mentioned inflammation in the first chapter, but we didn't talk much about how it works. Let's do that now.

To understand what inflammation does, let's use a metaphor. Have you ever organized a closet or a desk? How did that process go? You probably first made a huge mess that took over the entire room before organizing and putting everything away in its proper place. Simplistically, inflammation works the same way. An area that needs attention creates an immune response of increased blood flow, break down of damaged tissue, and various hormone releases all around the problem area until things are ready to go back to their normal, functioning status. The symptoms of inflammation—increased fluid (swelling, mucus), increased blood flow (warmth, heat, pain), increased immune response (puss, scabs), and increased hormones (more pain, fluid, blood flow, and immune response) are all good! The symptoms that we try to control and stop are created by your body as the way to heal and clean up. These are not symptoms of disease, but of healing.

When we stop the inflammatory process, we stop the body in the middle of its work. Let's look at an example of how this plays out. We can take certain medications to control symptoms, like many over the counter pain medications, called Cox-inhibitors. These medications shut down the cyclooxygenase (cox) enzyme, which in turn decreases symptoms we are experiencing, like swelling and pain. However, the cox enzyme not only initiates the inflammatory process, it also stops it. When we inhibit cox, we stop the symptoms, but we also stop the body's ability to resolve the inflammation. The result: low levels of inflammation that persist for a long time. Even if this inflammation is not easily noticeable through symptoms, it will take a toll on the body[1,4,6].

Cleaning up Old Messes

So inflammation is a necessary part of our body's protection against toxins. It is an amazing cleaner! If we want to heal, we need to allow this process to unfold unhindered. Also, as the body has backlogged cleaning work to do, you may experience increased amount of this cleaning process during your GAPS journey. This is a good sign! When the body is able to, it will clean up those areas of low-level inflammation, or remove stored toxins and repair the damage left behind. This means making a mess. If you had unresolved joint inflammation, for example, the immune system may initiate full-blown inflammation to clean it up, even if the original injury was years ago. Let it happen. If you allow the process to run its natural course (and the right nutritional building-blocks are present), at the end you should experience healing, and that joint may even feel as good as new!

Inflammation is used for more than physical injury. Toxins released by invading bacteria or viruses, heavy metals and other toxins from our bad gut flora, and allergens from foods or our environment can also cause the in-flammatory response to be initiated. In these cases, it is important to let the body do what it does best—clean up. When we are sick with a cold or the flu, don't stop the symptoms. Instead, rest and let the body fully dispose of the problem. When the body is cleaning up the toxins in a dusty corner, we can support it nutritionally with meat stock and fermented cod liver oil. When allergies flare, we can eat foods high in arachidonic acid (such as duck and chicken eggs and liver) to give the body the tools it needs to recognize and respond properly to the allergen. The immune system is amazing, and when we hinder its work, we are only hurting ourselves.

Detoxification Pathways

Whether toxins enter our bloodstream from the gut, or are put there through the cleaning process of the immune system, they have to be processed by the body in order to be eliminated. This processing follows our detoxification pathway, and different types of toxins get processed in different ways. First, let's look at how healthy detoxification pathways should function. Then we will look at what happens when detox organs become overwhelmed. Finally, we will discuss some different ways to support the detoxification pathway in various ways and at various stages.

Simplified Detoxification Pathways

Now say we have a toxin loose. If the toxin is water-soluble, it will be absorbed into the bloodstream. It then flows into the liver, where some types of tox-ins are removed. These toxins are excreted back into the intestines in bile, or transported to the kidneys to eventually be excreted in urine. Any toxins still present in the bloodstream flow next to the lungs, and most, including the toxic gases, are eliminated here.

Now let's follow the journey of a fat-soluble toxin. These toxins may be absorbed into the bloodstream or into the lymph fluid. It would then travel to the lungs, where most are eliminated. Any remaining toxins then dump into the bloodstream and flow to the liver, where the rest should be removed and eliminated.

Detoxification Organs

Several of the organs in our body play a large role in detoxification. These are the liver, kidney and bladder, lungs and skin. Let's look at these organs, and what happens when they stop functioning optimally.

Liver

Let's look more closely at the liver. An amazing organ, the liver filters an average of 1.45 liters of blood a minute[2]. As we discussed, toxins are not stored in the liver. As they are removed from the blood, they are either sent to the kidneys, or combined with bile and excreted into the intestines. There are two major detoxification pathways, or phases that the liver uses. Each phase is complex, and requires certain enzymes, vitamins, minerals, hormones and other substances to complete. Many people with GAPS do not have the requirements for these pathways to function well. This, combined with the large amount of toxins present, causes the liver to become overwhelmed. Its performance becomes poor, and many toxins are not removed from the blood, passing instead to the lungs and beyond.

Kidneys and Bladder

Kidneys also work hard, filtering the blood at a rate of 120-150 quarts a day. They combine these wastes with those they received from the liver into a liquid consisting largely of urea. This liquid is then stored in the bladder until it is eliminated[5]. When there are too many toxins, or they are too concentrated (in the case of dehydration), the liquid can irritate the kidneys or bladder, and can cause kidney infections, nephritis, chronic cystitis, bed wetting, bladder infections, and other related problems.

Supporting the Liver and Kidneys

The most obvious way to support these organs is to decrease the number of toxins they need to process. It is also important to provide a nutrient-dense diet, which will provide what these organs need to repair and perform. Doing the gentle detoxification activities discussed in chapter 2 are essential to relieve the toxic stress on these organs. Other methods of supporting these organs, like beet kvass, water with minerals, and juicing are discussed further on in this chapter.

Lungs

Most people do not know the lungs are a detox organ, let alone one of the most important ones! Toxic gases, along with some fat-soluble toxins, are eliminated through the lungs. Toxins are trapped in mucus and driven upward through ciliary action to be removed from the body. When the liver is not functioning well, or if the lungs are otherwise overwhelmed by toxins, damage occurs in the lung tissue. The body responds quickly, wanting to repair the damage. It initiates a bronchospasm, which closes off the small section of lung until it is repaired, often within 10-30 minutes. We experience this as chest tightness and shortness of breath (also known as an asthma attack). When we inhibit this bronchospasm with anti-asthmatic drugs, we again inhibit the body's ability to heal. The next time that damage occurs, both areas of damaged lung will be closed off in a spasm, so the body can repair them. If we continue to intervene, this pattern repeats itself until a large part of the lung becomes closed off. At this point the asthma is life-threatening, and may even lead to death[1].

Supporting the Lungs

In the case of asthma or other lung conditions, we can support our lungs in several ways. First, we need to stop the influx of toxins. We need to remove scents, cleaning fumes, and other manmade toxins from our environment. We also need to stop hindering the body in its repair work. If you or your child experiences shortness of breath, the person should sit still, be kept warm and calm, and take small sips of water from a teaspoon. The shortness of breath should pass within thirty minutes. No steroids or bronchodilators should be started. However, if the person is already using asthma medications, they need to slowly wean off. This should be done cautiously and under supervision, because the lungs may be so damaged that an untreated bronchospasm would be life threatening. Seek advice from your GAPS practitioner and prescribing provider to safely remove these medications. In the meantime, we can provide the lungs with healing and soothing nutrients in the form of fat. The lungs love fat, especially animal fat! If there is any lung damage, fats like butter should be consumed extensively. Finally, we can support the normal detox mechanism by performing deep breathing exercises. Simple breathing exercises cleanse and strengthen the lungs. Do these once or twice a day when you are calm and relaxed, not during a period of shortness of breath. Exercise also strengthens the lungs because it encourages deep breathing.

Skin

The skin's primary function is protection and defense, but it is also a detox organ. When other organs are overwhelmed, the skin can assist in detox. It especially helps the kidney with its detox load, since it is able to eliminate the same types of toxins. There is an enzyme in the skin that metabolizes toxins and converts them to crystals, including uric acid and urea. These crystals are then removed through pores as sweat. To help this process, it is important to stay hydrated and to induce sweating. You can induce sweating through activity and exercise, saunas, hot baths, and other activities that cause hyperthermia (fever). The skin can also become overwhelmed with toxins. If certain toxins are removed through sweat, if large amounts of toxins are removed, or if the skin cells are unhealthy, rashes can appear. These rashes are usually located near the site of the toxins or in areas that sweat more. They can also appear where the skin has been damaged by a burn, sun exposure, abrasion, or other area of weakness.

Rashes and Other Skin Eruptions

Rashes can be confusing to figure out. On one hand, a rash shows an unhealthy detox system and body full of toxins. For example, a rash may appear after you eat a certain food, signaling that you still have healing work to do, and to continue avoiding that food. On the other hand, it can show a healthy and healing body. For example, if steps are being taken toward better health, and the rash had improved for a while, its presence may mean that stored toxins are being removed from the body, a sign of improving health.

I recommend treating any skin eruptions as only one clue about what's going on. If you overall feel better, don't be discouraged by a worsening rash. But if you notice that every time you eat avocados you get a rash the next day, then there is something your body is not handling well and you may want to avoid avocados for a while. Skin eruptions are very common when experiencing a die-off reaction (see the next chapter), in which case you should reduce or stop the offending food or probiotic for a time.

Other Detox Methods

Near the beginning of this book, we discussed ways to detox while putting little to no strain on our detox organs. These are detox baths or footbaths, sunbathing, oil pulling, enemas and swimming in natural waters. Go back and review them if you need to. Because of the large number of toxins, it is important to support your body with these methods until your gut is cleaned up and your detox pathways are functioning better. You will find that some feel better to you then others. Allow your body to communicate with you about what types of detox are most helpful, and when. You will probably need to detox a lot in the beginning of your healing journey. As toxins are cleaned out, and your body's systems are functioning better, you will need to use these methods less and less.

Supporting Your Body's Detox Patterns

In a normal circadian rhythm, the body is concentrated on cleansing from 4am-10am every day. We also know that the immune system (inflammation) is more active at night, and hormones like growth hormone (which repairs damaged tissue in adults) are released in greater numbers while we are sleeping[6]. As always, we want to work with the body and support its normal patterns and rhythms. Sleep in warm blankets, but in a cool room, preferably with fresh air. It is important to get enough sleep and, if possible, not get up too early (unless you naturally wake up). Unless you suffer from adrenal fatigue, low blood sugar, or have recently started the GAPS protocol, you probably won't be hungry right when you wake up. The morning is a great time to just drink water, freshly pressed juices, and liver tonics. When you start feeling hungry, or around 10am, you should eat breakfast, as hunger is your body's signal that it is moving on from a cleansing focus. In addition to working with your body's rhythms, there are other things you can do to support detoxification in your body.

Fat

As we discussed with the lungs, fat plays an important role in detoxification. Not only does fat provide nutrients that repair damaged tissue, fat itself contains molecules that can be used for detoxification. This includes both animal and plant fats. Plant fats should be in the form of cold-pressed oils, and it is important to know the source and processing of the oils. Rancid, mixed or heated plant oils do not help with detoxing. In fact they are full of toxins themselves, adding to the overall toxic burden of the body. Therefore they should be avoided.

Water

We all know that we should drink water. Among other things, water is important for detoxification. The water that you drink should be filtered, at least through a carbon filter, to remove the chlorine and major contaminants. It is good to drink a full glass of warm or room-temperature water first thing in the morning. A little freshly-squeezed lemon juice and some added minerals will add to the detoxification effect. After that, water should be taken throughout the day only as desired. Too much water can lead to an electrolyte imbalance or hinder the absorption of your food. Listen to what your body needs. Drink water when you first start feeling thirsty, and you should drink only enough so that your urine is a very light shade of yellow. If it is dark yellow, you are not getting enough water. If it is clear, it is too diluted and you need more minerals. If your body is concentrating on cleansing, you may to desire more water than usual. On these days, make sure you are also taking in additional minerals in the form of real salt or mineral drops to balance out the increased water intake.

Minerals and Salt

On the GAPS protocol, it is recommended to get most of your water in the form of meat stock, freshly pressed juices, and fermented liquids. These liquids already have added minerals, so they help your body maintain a proper electrolyte balance. If you do drink water, keep in mind that you need to balance it out with minerals. One way to do this is by adding a little sea salt or a mineral drop or two to every glass of water. Not everyone prefers the taste of this, and it is acceptable to get your minerals at a separate time from the water you drink. You can salt your food, take a single daily glass of water with several mineral drops, or lick salt off your hand. The idea is to give your body enough minerals to balance the water you are drinking.

When I talk about real salt, I am talking about unrefined sea salt. These salts contain iodine and all the other minerals that naturally come in it. The three salts with the highest mineral content are Celtic sea salt, Real Salt (from Utah) and Himalayan sea salt (in descending order). You can find the ones I use on the resource page on my website.

Have you ever felt like the water you are drinking is dry and doesn't satisfying your thirst? That was your body signaling you that it needs minerals, not just water. If that happens, try adding in those minerals, as we discussed. If you find yourself drinking and urinating excessively, you probably need more minerals. These minerals are also needed for detox so make sure you are giving your body enough of a supply.

Liver Tonics

Liver tonic refers to a group of fermented beverages that have specific detoxification action in the liver and blood. There are several beverages that meet this criteria, but the most common is beet kvass. Kvass simply means beverage, so beet kvass is exactly what it says it is—a beet beverage. It is made of three simple ingredients—cubed beets, sea salt, and water. It is left on the counter to ferment, and then a small amount of it is to be drunk daily. As with all ferments, start out slowly and watch for die-off symptoms. It is best drunk on an empty stomach (30 min before meals, or 2 hrs after meals), and can be combined with freshly pressed juices if desired. Work your way up slowly to the recommended dose of 4 ounces two times a day. Beets have incredible cleansing properties, both in the liver and to the blood, and should be consumed daily.

Egg Whites

While egg yolks are mostly cholesterol, the protein in egg whites is largely cleansing, especially if consumed raw. And I mean real egg whites, not the highly-process protein powders you can buy. Early on in GAPS, egg whites may not be well tolerated. This is why they are left out of stage 2, and why they are first introduced in a cooked form. When tolerated, raw egg whites can be consumed to assist with detoxification. This can be easily done in the delicious GAPS milkshake. You can find this recipe in the GAPS book, or on my website. It is a smoothie made of freshly pressed juices, fat (usually sour cream), raw egg, and honey if desired. It is also a liver tonic, and many people consume this daily as their first meal in the morning, as it is fairly sustaining, and quickly digested and absorbed. It is great for detoxing, and also as an on-the-go meal.

Plants

Plants are very important in cleansing! As discussed in the previous chapter, we are going to generally refer to plants as cleansing rather than building. While plants do contain vitamins, minerals, and bioflavonoids, we get the most benefit from the cleansing properties of fiber, antioxidants, enzymes, and other detoxifying substances. In the last chapter we discussed cooking vegetables to assist in the digestion and absorption of nutrients. However, when tolerated, eating raw vegetables is also important. Raw plants are not introduced until later in the Intro diet. This is largely due to the difficulty in digesting fiber. When the intestines are inflamed and irritated, fiber can act like sandpaper, further irritating the gut wall. Until this resolves, someone may be able to tolerate raw plants that have had much of the fiber removed, such as in juicing.

Freshly Pressed Juices

Juicing is the process of separating and removing a significant amount of the fiber present in fruits, vegetables, and other edible plants. It has been used for centuries to treat disease, and is a gentle and efficient way to cleanse the body. There are many different recipes that can be used for juicing, and different combinations will provide support for varying problems, as well as different mixes of nutrients and flavors. There are many recipe books about juicing, so we will not discuss that here. The fruits, vegetables, and herbs used for juicing should be organic and fresh. It is best to have at least 50% therapeutic ingredients, but flavor is important, especially for children, so there is no problem in adding sweeter ingredients such as fruit to make it taste good!

Because of their properties, it is recommended to have a small amount of beet, cabbage, and ginger in your mix. Be careful—a little beet goes a long way! There are mixed opinions on raw spinach, so I generally don't recommend for spinach to be juiced or eaten raw.

You can drink these juices on their own, or add them to a GAPS milkshake. You could also add your liver tonic to the juice, or drink it at the same time. It is best to consume juices immediately after making, because it will begin to oxidize soon after it is separated from the fiber. Depending on your type of juicer, how you store it, and what ingredients you use, it may keep up to 72 hours without losing much nutritional benefit.

As mentioned before, it is best to drink the juice first thing in the morning. If able, it is beneficial to drink another batch of freshly pressed juices in the middle of the afternoon, again on an empty stomach. If this is not possible, go ahead and juice! Juicing anytime is better than not juicing at all. And, as always, listen to what your body needs. Some people see a lot of benefit from juicing, while others only notice a little difference. If your body responds well, make it a priority to juice every day.

A Note on Fasting

There are times when fasting may be an appropriate action to improve health. If you feel that you should fast, I recommend that you consult with a GAPS practitioner or other natural health provider. Fasts longer than 72 hours should never be undertaken without direct supervision from someone who is familiar with fasting. For most people with GAPS, rebuilding takes priority over cleansing, and they can hardly go 3 hours between meals. This is normal, and you should listen to your body and eat as often as it prompts you to eat.

There may be times when your body asks for a short fast, maybe skipping a meal or two, or even going an entire day without eating. This is more likely to happen further into the protocol, sometimes during a cleansing period such as an illness, or after an enema. If that is the case, you can cautiously listen to your body and abstain from food for a short period of time. If, during that time, you become dizzy, disoriented, or significantly weak, you need to eat something. Sometimes you don't feel like eating because you are bored of your food options, or you are only offering your body foods it doesn't want or need. Try finding a new recipe, or give your body more options, because in this case your body is not cleansing, it wants to eat!

Juice Fasting

Juice fasts are not ever recommended without supervision and guidance. They can be appropriate later, especially if symptoms are primarily from toxin overload. But any type of fast—juice, vegan, water, or otherwise—should always be done with direct supervision from a professional. Knowing how to start and stop the fast (as well as how long to continue and what to eat) may need to be individualized, and can result in harm if done incorrectly.

Chapter Six

The last area we need to discuss is the residents in our neighborhood. They consist of bacteria, viruses, worms, parasites, amoebas, yeasts, fungi, and other microorganisms. Each person has an individual mix of residents, although they usually resemble those of their parents. But before we get into this, let's take a (very) quick look into the history of bacteria discovery.

History of Bacteria Discovery

Bacteria was first seen in the 1670's by Antonie van Leeuwenhoek, but it was not widely studied until the late 1800's, most famously by Louis Pasteur[2]. Since then, mainstream science has studied bacteria and other microorganisms through the lens of this Germ theory, based on the premise that these tiny life forms should be avoided and destroyed in order to preserve health. Although this theory continues to be the most popular, another theory, the Cellular theory, may better explain our relationship with microorganisms. Antoine Bechamp, alive at the same time as Pasteur, was a large contributor to the Cellular theory, which has been largely rejected by the science and medical communities. The cellular theory asserts that disease is caused by the activity of bacteria in the presence of already diseased or dead tissue. According to this theory, those same bacteria in a healthy environment pose no threat of poor health. We can see an example of this in nature. Wood does not rot when it is healthy and alive, but only after it is diseased or dead. The Cellular theory claims that it is the same in our bodies, and that the microbes in our body only act on tissue that is already diseased or dead. Some say that even Pasteur, at the end of his life, believed the Cellular theory to be more correct than his own Germ theory[4]. The debate continues quietly but extensively in the scientific community, and you can read many articles and books about this if you so choose. I personally find everything I learn about this topic fascinating.

All right, enough with the history lesson! In order to understand how probiotics are beneficial to us, we need to adjust our perspective. A strict belief in the Germ theory does not allow for the presence of good bacteria. In reality, we now know there are good bacteria that live inside us. So I invite you to open your perspective a little, and entertain the ideas of the Cellular theory. Increasingly, the study of the human body has shown a helpful, symbiotic relationship between our cells and the cells of other microorganisms, known as the human microbiome.

The Human Microbiome

To review, the human microbiome is a symbiotic colony of bacteria, yeast, virus, and other microorganisms that live in and on our bodies. We don't know every interaction that occurs, but we do know that these bacteria and other microorganisms (referred to as our flora) play some important roles. Our flora is passed on to us from our parents, but it will change depending on what we are exposed to and what our body needs to adapt to[3]. While the functions of this flora are described with a focus on the gut, many of them are occurring throughout the whole body.

Roles of the Human Microbiome

1. Maintain the integrity of the gut lining. The flora plays a major role in keeping the lining functional and structurally correct. Without proper flora, the enterocytes that line the gut wall are unable to reproduce properly, and the gut flora helps the gut tissue adapt to different needs.
2. Digest and absorb food. The gut flora produces enzymes that allow us to break down our food and absorb the helpful nutrients our body needs to function. Some foods are indigestible to us without the help of certain bacteria. Without healthy flora, we are not able to absorb what we need from food or even supplements, and we become malnourished.
3. Produce vitamins and minerals for our body. We have discovered that healthy gut flora actually synthesizes nutrients we need, such as vitamin K2, folic acid, many of the B vitamins, and others. They release these vitamins as the body needs them, to be absorbed into the bloodstream and used by the body.
4. Communicate with the immune system. We already discussed this in a previous chapter, but I will list it again here. Healthy gut flora plays a vital role in proper immune system functioning, protecting against invading species as well as communicating with the body what things are foods, preventing the development of allergies.
5. Help regulate our metabolism. All the research about the human microbiome is fairly new, but scientists are beginning to link the presence of certain bacteria to a healthier body type and less incidence of disease, and other bacteria to obesity and disease.
6. Prevent overpopulation of opportunistic or pathogenic flora. Even the most healthy person has small amounts of gut flora living inside them that could cause disease, but the good flora make sure that they never get out of hand. This occurs everywhere in our body—in the gut, the lungs and other mucous membranes, the skin, and all throughout our bodies. One example of this is Candida albicans. This fungus causes many unpleasant symptoms, but it also performs tasks that are helpful to the body, such

as eating dead tissue. Therefore, it is to the body's benefit to allow a small amount of it to be present.

7. Neutralize toxins and remove them from the body. A major role of our flora is to identify and bind to toxins that come into contact with our body. If the flora is unable to neutralize the substance, it will continue to cling to that substance, preventing it from entering our bloodstream, until it has been eliminated from the body[1].

We are discovering more about this amazing human microbiome all the time. You can read more about this in the book, *Gut and Psychology Syndrome*, or other published research. We may never know all the symbiotic relationships formed between our bodies and our microbiome, but we do know that we cannot live without them!

Inviting Better Tenants

We are finally to the main purpose of this chapter—discussing the residents! When healing GAPS, most people need to do a major eviction and resettlement of the current residents of the body. But how? As we discussed in the previous two chapters, we first need to start changing the environment. If you want to keep good tenants, you have to have working appliances and strong walls! Making these changes will begin to put the pressure on pathogenic and opportunistic bacteria to either clean up their act or get out.

At the same time, you need to introduce beneficial bacteria to the mix. There are two ways to do this—through probiotic capsules or powder, and with the use of fermented foods. Healthy gut flora contains a wide mixture of microorganisms, which may vary from person to person. Different mixes of probiotics, and different ferments, introduce a variety of strains, some of which will take up residence in your body, first in your gut, then spread everywhere else.

How to Choose a Probiotic

Choosing a probiotic can be difficult. There are so many to choose from, and they all claim to be the best. Some claim to be the best because of their many strains, other because they only have a few. So which one do you choose? In her book, Dr. Campbell-McBride makes some suggestions for choosing a probiotic. First, she recommends that you choose a probiotic from a company that has researched, proven claims. Second, that the company should test every batch and be willing to present that data. Third, the formulation you take should contain as many strains as possible of Lactobacilli, Bifidobacteria, and various soil bacterium. Fourth, the concentration should be at least 8 billion bacterial cells per gram. (Dosage depends on the age of the person, as well as their health status. You will want to start with a low dose, and work up to a therapeutic dose. This could be 2-20 billion bacterial cells per day, depending. After a period of time, the dose should be reduced to a maintenance dose, which is determined on an individual basis[1].)

Probiotic powder or capsules can be thought of as troops. When you are in a war (which is happening inside your body, especially when you are first starting GAPS) you have to send in many fresh troops. For most people who suffer from GAPS, it would be impossible to eat enough fermented and cultured food to provide the numbers of probiotic "troops" they need. Probiotic supplements allow us to send in the millions of troops we need each day. They also allow us to know and control the dose, which is necessary to manage die-off symptoms (discussed later in the chapter).

Fermentation

Fermenting foods is an ancient practice, when its primary purpose was to preserve food in the absence of refrigeration. With the onset of refrigeration, we have gotten away from this tradition, which has added to the problems caused by our modern diet. But fermenting still lives! The knowledge and practice of this tradition continue, not only in traditional societies, but in the kitchens of modern people as well. There are many resources and recipes related to fermentation, so we will not discuss that here. But what we will discuss is the benefit of these ferments, especially in the way of providing a wonderful and diverse mixture of probiotics!

Fermentation, simply, is creating an environment for good, beneficial bacteria to grow while inhibiting the growth of bad, pathogenic bacteria (sound familiar?). This is done with salt. Vegetables (or other foods) are put in salt-water brine, which kills bad bacteria, molds, and other undesirable microbes, but does not harm beneficial ones. In this environment, lactic-acid producing bacteria (LABs) and other helpful microbes flourish and multiply, eventually able to protect themselves from any bad microbes. This is called wild fermentation. To ensure a correct environment, or to speed up the process, we can do lacto-fermentation. This process entails adding our own LABs in the form of whey, probiotic powder, or culture starter packets. This "stacks the deck," further guaranteeing that only beneficial probiotics will be allowed to grow.

Each vegetable has an individual profile of probiotics (including soil bacterium) living in and on it. When we ferment a variety of vegetables, we are ingesting different bacteria species. For this reason it is important to consume a variety of fermented vegetables, as well as cultured dairy products (if tolerated), in your daily diet.

Culturing Dairy

The process of culturing dairy is similar, and uses the presence of LABs to prevent putrefaction of milk. Instead, the milk or cream is cultured, and the presence of beneficial probiotics prevents the growth of spoiling microbes, allowing the dairy product to keep longer. Examples of this are sour cream (creme fraische), yogurt, cultured butter, and kefir. Some of these can be store-bought if processed correctly, but most can be simply and less expensively made at home.

Kombucha and Water Kefir

Just a note on other types of fermented foods and beverages. It is possible to ferment just about anything, from meat and legumes to SCOBYs and kefir grains. But some ferments are not as beneficial to you right now. Kombucha and water kefir, for example, are easily overrun by yeast and there is usually some leftover sugar. I don't recommend introducing these, or fermented fruits, until you are at least on stage 5 (or even later) and tolerating fruit sugar well. Not only will you be less likely to react at this time, you will also be more likely to recognize if your body has any reaction to any sugar contained in these beverages. If you have any reaction, then you know you are not ready for that food or drink yet.

Die-Off Reaction

When taking probiotics, it is common to experience a die-off, or Herxheimer reaction. This is essentially a detox reaction caused from the toxins released by the bad flora when it dies. The toxins, each one causing symptoms in the body, are suddenly released from the exploding microbe, and cause a temporary increase in those symptoms. This reaction can be severe, and for this reason it is important to start any new probiotic, ferment, or cultured dairy product slowly and cautiously. However, it is also good news, because it means that the neighborhood is changing!

But more is not better. A toxin release that is too fast can cause additional problems, or cause healing to be slower. And if the body isn't ready to support the new environment, the body will revert to its earlier state. If the residents change faster than the environment, they won't stay around. This will only result in money wasted on probiotics, and time wasted being miserable. Instead, approach this resettlement at a slow and steady pace. This prevents probiotic waste, sets an appropriate pace for healing, and allows the body to keep up with the toxins being released, largely preventing them from doing additional damage or causing symptoms.

Anything that is killing bad bacteria can potentially cause a die-off reaction. This includes consuming meat stock or fresh-pressed juices, eating certain foods or avoiding others, being in the sun too long, taking detox baths, or taking a certain supplement. These reactions are no reason to stop—they are good news—but if you experience them it is a good idea to slow down or stop whatever you think is causing the reaction and allow things to settle down before continuing. When you restart that thing again, begin with a very small amount and gradually work your way up, listening to what your body can handle. This start and stop pace can seem pointless, but nothing good is ever wasted. You cannot regulate the timing of your "advancement," only your body can. Be patient and let your body direct this timeline.

Topical Probiotics

The gut is the breeding ground of our body's flora, so most of our focus is taking in probiotics, in whatever form, orally. This is an inside-out approach. However, we can populate our body using an outside-in approach too! This is helpful in the case of skin eruptions, yeast overgrowth, ear or sinus problems, incorrect bladder, vaginal or anal flora, and other things of this nature. This can be done using a probiotic food or mixture, such as sour cream (my favorite), yogurt or milk kefir, tallow+probiotic powder, or things like this. Because these are only foods, you cannot overdose on them when you are putting them on your skin, so apply as often as necessary. They may cause a slight detox reaction, in which case you should take a break for a day or so to allow the inflammation to do its work of cleaning before continuing to apply, as necessary.

It's a Beautiful Day in the Neighborhood

The goal of this resettlement of your gut (and eventually your entire body) is to establish the environment you have worked so hard to create. Even with all the right structures and building blocks, a 5-star neighborhood will go downhill if you don't have the right people living there. This is true in your body, and that is why probiotics are so important. Remember all the amazing things that our flora does for us? If they aren't living with us, we will quickly go right back to where we started. So start getting your probiotics, make a good environment for them, and don't stop sending in fresh troops too early.

The information we have covered in the past three chapters are the core elements. In the next chapters we will talk about how to work with your body, and how to troubleshoot when things seem to be going wrong. Continue to grow your understanding of how and why each piece works in your body, and also don't forget to do them!

Chapter Seven

W hat does it mean to be an expert detective? In another online article, "One Man's Meat is Another Man's Poison", Dr. Campbell-McBride describes how to work with your body to understand what you need to eat, and when[1]. I like to describe this idea as being an expert detective, and that is what this chapter is all about. Let's talk about the steps that need to be taken to become an expert detective. They are listed below.

• Listen to your body and stop ignoring it
• Clean up the signals coming to your senses so you know which ones are real
• Become a partner with your body, giving it a say in what it needs, and when
• Learn what your body it trying to tell you with undesirable signals (symptoms)
• Learn how to avoid undesirable symptoms by what you heard it telling you

How to Listen

To become an expert detective, you need to first learn how to understand what your body is telling you. Then you need to listen to it! Most of us have declared to our body that it doesn't know what it is doing, and that we are in charge. We do this in pretty much every area of our lives. We eat when we want to, and what we want to. We ignore the pangs of hunger, and wait to eat because we are busy, or lazy, or trying to lose weight. We force ourselves to eat at certain times, even if we are not hungry. We may eat all that is on our plate because we don't want to waste the $20 we just spent in the restaurant, or we skip many meals altogether because we got caught up in our work. At times we satisfy our thirst with coffee or a soda instead of water, or drink water to curb our hunger. And it's not just limited to food. We also push ourselves to stay up late finishing a project because we are on a deadline, and then drag ourselves out of bed four hours later to get to work on time. We drink caffeine to stay awake, then take sleeping pills to go to sleep. We work when we are sick, or push through when we have a headache or other pain, often taking medications to mask our symptoms. Little by little, from the time we are children, we tell our bodies that they have no say in how they get treated. We dissolve the partnership that should exist between us.

Now, I understand that some of this is, unfortunately, unavoidable in our culture. But ask yourself how many of those decisions are really within your control? If you are not hungry for breakfast until 10 am, consider bringing something to work and take a break to eat it when your body is asking for it. Build the habit of turning off your TV and going to bed when you are tired. Avoid last-minute stress and deadlines by a little more discipline and a little less procrastination? For most of us, we could listen to our body a lot more than we do. By the way, I am not saying I am perfect in this—I still ignore my body, especially when it comes to sleep. But I have found that if I listen to my body, I feel much better. I have been most successful in re-establishing a partnership with my body in regard to mealtimes, and what it wants to eat. And I feel much better. Why? Because I am working with my body, instead of being in disharmony with it.

Why Listen?

The body's metabolism is constantly changing. Every hour, and sometimes every minute, it requires different things for its activity. Once you start listening to your body, it will tell you what it needs at that time. It uses primarily desire (or not) for certain foods, thirst, hunger, taste, and even smell. The body's normal, 24-hour circadian rhythm is divided into two main periods related to digestion, a cleansing period and a feeding period. Like we discussed previously, the cleansing period is between 4am and 10am. This is why many people are not hungry for breakfast early in the morning.

During the rest of the day, the body is potentially wanting fuel in the form of food. It will not be all the time, however, and if you listen, it will tell you when and what it wants you to eat. It may want different things throughout the day, or the food it wants may vary from day to day. Some days you may want to eat meat and stock all day long, but the next day you are happy with just carrots and water. When you first begin, you will likely find that the "rebuilding days" are more frequent, but that later on the "cleansing days" begin to happen more often.

Clean up the Signals

It is also important to eat the types of food that your body is wanting. This is accomplished first by getting rid of the processed foods in your diet. All processed foods have ingredients in them designed specifically to manipulate your taste buds, and most have known addictive ingredients in them so that you continue to buy and eat that food. Additionally, foods high in simple carbs or sugars feed and multiply flora, and those "bad guys" begin to override the signals your body is sending. For example, when you crave sugary foods, it is not your body asking for it, it is the "bad guys." As you eat foods, such as animal fats and meat stock, that are helpful only to your body and microbes that work with your body, you will begin to starve things like candida. As the false signals diminish, your body will be able to direct you to what foods are truly helpful to you!

Renewing the Partnership

As your body begins to send you stronger signals, it will communicate in the form of your senses, and your desire (or not) for certain foods. When you feel hungry, you should think "What do I want most to eat?" or, as Dr. Campbell-McBride says "What would I kill for right now?" Once you have thought of that food (and make sure it's not something like a jelly doughnut), then get that food and smell it. If it smells delicious, taste it. If it tastes delicious, then eat it! As you enjoy it, pay attention to how much your body wants of it. If you finish your portion and still want more, make some more. And when your stomach says "enough!" stop eating it, even if you only have a bite or two left on your plate. That extra bite may cause your body to work too hard, resulting in sluggishness, headache, brain fog, or other similar symptoms. It takes time to perfect this, so don't be too hard on yourself. But do pay attention. When you get a headache after eating, or feel that you need to lie down, your body is telling you something. Try to listen, try to figure out what it is telling you. Each time you understand why your body has reacted a certain way, you are becoming more and more of an expert detective! If you approach your body as a partner, instead of a pest, or even an enemy, you will be amazed at how successful you can be at feeling good! As with anything worth doing, it will take time, attention, and work to become proficient, but each victory will be noticeable and will bring benefit!

Undesirable Signals

Just as your body has a way to tell you what it needs, it can also tell you when something you do was not helpful to you. That symptom (signal) can come because of a food you shouldn't have eaten, or because you ate too much food, or didn't eat soon enough, or because it was the wrong food for that time. You get symptoms when you eat the wrong thing at the wrong time. I'll say that again. Your body creates a symptom because you gave it the wrong thing, too much of the right thing, or not enough of what it needed at that time. This is why it's so important to become an expert detective. Unless you plan on talking to your practitioner every day, even every minute, you need to learn what your body is asking for. Only you can hear what your body is asking, and only you can be the partner it needs to achieve what you both want—good health!

What are some of these undesirable signals? Your body uses things such as headaches and other pain, stomach upset or heaviness, nausea, loose stools, flatulence, indigestion, heartburn, skin irritation, sudden tiredness or brain fog, or an overall sensation of not feeling well. As you clear up the signal pathways, these symptoms come quickly, often immediately or within minutes. Pay attention to these signals! When you start experiencing them, stop what you are doing. Try to figure out what the symptom has come from, and adjust to accommodate what your partner, your body, is asking you to do.

Muted Signals

If these symptoms (signals) are ignored, then other symptoms will develop, and these are more difficult to decipher. Examples of these symptoms are acne, constipation, diarrhea, or both. (Also autoimmune disease, allergies, chronic pain, dark circles under the eyes, and so much more.) These things develop because your body can no longer keep up. It can no longer send you a signal that says "Hey, when you did that, I had to work hard to adjust and fix the damage. Just FYI, maybe you shouldn't do that again." Instead, you are getting a signal from all the parts of the body that are affected. It says "Ouch! Help! I am overwhelmed here and I can no longer function properly." As time goes on, that signal may get louder, or may get much quieter. If it gets quieter, it does not necessarily mean that it is fixed. If we listened closely, maybe we would hear this message "I guess no help is coming. I see that we are lacking vital supplies. I will just keep limping on here as long as I can. Send help if possible."

Signs of Healing

This is why, when you start healing, it seems like some symptoms are getting worse. When supplies start coming into the camp, those areas that have been quiet and just trying to hang on start demanding: "Hey! We need some help here! Don't forget about us!" This is good! It takes energy to ask and to rebuild, and when your body is getting to that stage, be encouraged! This is showing good progress on the reversal and repair of damage that has already been done. These times can be the most emotionally upsetting in your health journey, but they are good. When you experience these things, keep going— you are on the right track!

Take the Time to Prepare

Being prepared to give your body what it needs, when it needs it, takes some extra work and planning. You may begin getting a headache because you need to eat. But suppose you are out? You need to bring food with you so you can be prepared for what your body needs. Does this sound extreme? Is it really healthy to be catering to your body's every whim? I admit, in the beginning, it feels more like a one-way partnership. But think of this . . . you have been the demanding partner for most of your existence. So it makes sense that as you are finding a healthy balance and partnership, the partner that has been ignored may need a little more attention. When a lot of healing has occurred, you will find that you are able to wait a little while to eat without getting a headache, or find ways to get your body ready to eat earlier than usual if you really need to. As you heal, your partner, your body, will be able to be more flexible when it needs to be. But remember that your body is not your enemy. When it is sending you a signal, it is not to ruin your day or run your life. It wants the same thing that you do—to be productive and pain free. And because it knows what your body needs to best function, it will tell you, so you can do it.

A Healthy Body is a Quiet Body

For many of us, this is difficult to understand. We have become very used to our bodies making noise from pain, fatigue, or other things. We have forced our bodies into silence by ignoring signals for help (as we just discussed above), and we may think that if we start listening to our body, it will only get louder and more demanding. We can see our physical needs as a nuisance because they so often seem to get in the way of what we want to do. This is not true at all. A functional body is very quiet—willingly quiet. It wants to fade into the background so creativity, productivity, and love can outflow. This is our purpose, and our body wants to walk in that purpose as much as we do. It is only when there is trouble that it brings itself to conscious thought and physical feeling.

Think about a part of your body that doesn't hurt right now. Maybe it's your forearm, or the tip of your nose. Would you have thought about this point if you weren't choosing to? No, you wouldn't. Why not? Because there's nothing wrong with it. Unless you have a muscle cramp, or a bruise, or a broken bone, or some other thing that is wrong, that part of your body is quiet. The same is true of your body (and mind) as a whole. When it is working well, it is silent, going about its business with quiet efficiency. Again, it is only when something is wrong that your body begins to call attention to the part that needs help. And, as we discussed earlier, it will continue to make noise until it is either fixed, or it gets too worn out to continue calling for help.

How to Sort Through the Signals

If it's true that pain, discomfort, or other unpleasant signals are only present because something is wrong, then you may be very anxious to get started doing something about it. I'm sure you, like all of us, can think of many ways you are aware of your body, and are now worried about how many things need attention and repair. It isn't good to dwell on this feeling too long because it is easy to feel hopeless or paralyzed. But in this moment I want you to think deeper. I would urge you to get out a journal or a piece of paper to write down your thoughts about this. If you are using the My Daily Insights journal, there is room to do this exercise within the first few pages. I would encourage you to stop reading this right now, and do the exercise below.

Finding Your Why

Think about your body crying out for help. How does that make you feel? The purpose of this exercise is to find your "Why." To be successful on the long and difficult journey of healing that you are likely facing, you need to hold on to why you are on the journey in the first place. What is it that you want? What do you care about? Why is all of this worth it? What will be better on the other end if you persist on this journey?

OK, great, you have written out your Why (if you haven't done the exercise above yet, stop right now and do it!). Now let's talk about what you can do. Especially if you are not particularly in tune with your body right now, it may seem like an overwhelming task to listen, understand, and follow the signals that your body is sending. How are you going to accomplish this? The same way you eat an elephant—one bite at a time. Continue to re-read this chapter, going through the steps to becoming an expert detective one at a time. Practice! Try to listen, try to understand. Every time you try, you will get a little bit better. Each time, you and your partner will learn how to understand each other a little better, and that communication will get a little more efficient. This requires a lot of patience, especially with yourself. You will mess up many times! That's okay! Keep trying, it will get easier.

Getting Started

Even if you aren't a super detective yet, you can still start healing your body. That is the beautiful thing about what Dr. Campbell-McBride has discovered and laid out in the GAPS protocol. Even before you understand your body's signals to you, you can start making healing progress. As a general rule, there are some foods that are helpful to the body, and some foods that are harmful to the body. You can start moving forward by eating the good and helpful foods that are discussed in this book, and avoiding those that are harmful (or at least unhelpful) to the body. You can begin to get strong and heal, even while you are developing your partnership and detective skills.

Start Today!

In this chapter, we have discussed why it's important to listen to your body, and how to clean up the channels coming from your body so you can understand what your body is communicating to you. You can learn to understand when your body is asking for help, and how to work with your body to give it the things it needs to accomplish what you both want—good health. And you can start now! You can begin to develop a beautiful partnership with your body that will work to serve you for the rest of your life.

Chapter Eight

The Purpose of this Chapter

This chapter is to help you look deeper into troublesome symptoms you may be experiencing. It is built on principles found in other chapters, and I would encourage you to read those chapters first. For example, if you don't understand what meat stock does in your body, there are answers in this chapter that won't make as much sense. If you have read this book straight through, I hope you already have some ideas about why you feel like you are getting worse. But sometimes it is beyond your level of "detective rank." If you are at a loss about what to do, try walking through this chapter, analyzing the questions and suggestions to see which ones may apply to you in this situation. They are written in the order that I ask them in, and I suggest you follow that order as well.

Review What You are Eating

Whenever you start feeling worse, physically or emotionally, you should look first at what you are eating (or not eating). Again, there is no magic formula meal plan. If anything, the "magic formula" is to listen to your body (more details in the previous chapter) and give it what it is asking for. If you are still new to listening to your body, or if you can't quite figure out what it is telling you (it still happens to me occasionally), consider one of the following directions.

• **You are not eating enough fat.** This is often the culprit, and what I recommend people address first. In most cases, you should be eating at least ½ cup of added animal fat daily, if not much more. Maybe you were eating enough previously, but eating fat can be a full-time job, so you may have slacked off a bit. Or maybe you were not eating enough in the first place.

• **You are not consuming enough meat stock.** This is another daily habit that is vital, but difficult to keep up. There are many ideas about how to do this in chapter four.

• **You are eating too much fermented food.** While it is possible that the problem comes from you not eating enough fermented foods, more often people get into trouble because they are eating too much, and experiencing unpleasant die-off symptoms. You should have at least a little fermented food with each meal, but in the beginning, that may mean a small spoonful or less. If you think this may be your issue, decrease your intake to a liquid spoonful of one fermented food with each meal (less if you need to) for a few days. If symptoms subside or lessen, then this was likely your imbalance.

- **You are not drinking enough to detox.** This may mean that you are not juicing enough, or that you need to drink more water. Toxin build-up symptoms look a lot like die-off symptoms (because die-off is a type of detox reaction), or may be a headache, tinnitus, increased sensitivity, decreased stress tolerance (including noise and environment, emotional reaction, or cold temperature).

- **You are eating too much sugar.** Natural sugars count in this! In this case, "too much" is highly subjective, and depends on what is going on in your body. I have found that sugar generally affects mood the most. If you are experiencing moodiness and cannot figure out why, try removing all natural sugars (or returning to Intro Stage 3). After a few days, look for any positive change. If you *have* sugar cravings that last longer than 24 hours, then there is likely something (a "bad guy") that is controlling your taste for sugar. If that's the case, you need to remove sugar for at least a couple weeks in an attempt to starve those sugar cravers out. If you *don't* experience cravings after removing sugar, and you're not sure if your moods were affected, try eating some natural sugar and see how your body reacts. If you notice an increase in moodiness, often within a few hours, then your body has (wrongly) become dependent on that natural sugar. Remove it for at least a couple weeks before trying to add it back in.

- **You need to properly prepare your nuts and seeds.** Nuts and seeds need to be properly prepared before they become digestible. This is accomplished by soaking, sprouting or fermenting them. Directions on how to properly prepare seeds can be readily found online or in *Nourishing Traditions*.

- **You are cheating too much!** Again, "cheating" is going to mean something different for every person. For some people, "cheating" is going to mean that they eat pizza, or drink a soda. For others it means that they ate something on a stage higher than where they are. And for some, it may mean that they skipped their meat stock for the day, or they ate two apples instead of one. I define "cheating" as ignoring your body (it may be accidental) and eating something that is not good for it *at that time*. Remember, *at this time* is very important. There are many foods that are good, and will be good for you later, but *right now* it is not helpful to your body. And, during healing, anything that is not helpful to your body is harmful to your body. When you are in the intense healing period during the GAPS protocol, any unnecessary energy used to digest less-then-helpful food is going to slow your healing progress. You simply do not have any extra energy, so save it for what your body is prioritizing—healing. Soon you will need to heal less, and you will have the energy to digest more complicated foods.

- **You are doing things out of habit, not because your body is requesting it.** It is not uncommon to suddenly stop tolerating a food for a period of time. I have gone through periods where I suddenly started reacting to foods that I had been eating for a long time without problems. One time, for about 3 months, I would get extremely irritable if I ate any form of sugar, even in fruit. Another time, for about a month, I would get nauseated and a headache if I ate eggs. Each intolerance that developed also ended. I was able to eat those foods again, after something in my body changed (some I have figured out, others I haven't). Don't eat a food over and over again just because it's "what you do." Your body's needs can change, and if you are not paying attention, your disharmony can cause discomfort.

Review How Much You are Cleansing

The importance of detoxing cannot be stressed enough! When you are not helping your body remove toxins, you will likely notice that your thinking is clouded, you may have disrupted sleep, headaches, or generally feel worn out, sore, or moody. When someone "just feels bad" but can't really pinpoint what is wrong, my first thought is that they have too many toxins. To clarify, I am talking about toxins that are hanging around in the bloodstream, ones that the body is trying to flush out. Everyone may have a lot of toxins encapsulated in our fat cells, but they don't cause many active symptoms. The body stored them for this very purpose—they cause limited damage stored in a fat cell, as opposed to being free to roam around the body.

Remember, part of GAPS is having damaged detox pathways, so it's safe to assume that the body needs help dealing with the toxins that are present. If you are struggling with indistinct, vague, or subtle symptoms, try spending more time detoxing. This can be in the form of detox baths, oil pulling, sunbathing, enemas, drinking more water, or juicing. Different people respond differently to different methods, so pay attention. You may find that sunbathing leaves you feeling worse, while detox baths energize you. Do the things that make you feel better! While there may be a time and place for inducing a large toxin release in your body, now is not the time! Your body is already overwhelmed (that's why you are having symptoms). Help it clean up, so it can focus on healing. Cleaning happens later—and often so slowly that you won't even notice it happening.

Note on Chelation Therapy

When someone has a known toxin exposure, especially if a heavy metal is involved, the topic of chelation therapy often comes up. Chelation therapy is designed to remove heavy metals and minerals from the body by injecting chemicals into the bloodstream. There are mixed views on this practice. The main concerns about chelation therapy are that it will be done improperly and without proper support to the body. This can actually increase (sometimes dramatically) the symptoms someone is experiencing. This is not only miserable, but at times the flood of toxins from the release causes deep or permanent damage to the liver, kidneys, or other organs. Except in rare cases, the reason there are so many toxins in the body is because the body can't detox! Chelation therapy often works with the body's normal detox pathways, which aren't functioning well. This is why chelation therapy, especially early in the GAPS protocol, can be damaging. Dr. Campbell-McBride does not recommend chelation therapy in most instances, and she has found that when lab work is done, patients who have been on the GAPS protocol for 6-12 months without any specific chelation therapy have significantly reduced levels of the toxins that were overwhelming their body. I think of it in this simple way: the body wants to be clean. If it hasn't removed something it's because the body is unable, not unwilling. When we give it the support it needs to function properly, health will be restored to the body.

Evaluate your Environment and Lifestyle

If you are experiencing symptoms you can't figure out, think about your life as a whole. Have you recently moved or changed office environments? Redecorated? Changed detergent? Got a new pet? Is it a different season? Do you have different circumstances or stressors in your life? Did you recently introduce a new food or ferment, or change probiotics? Were you recently ill, or have you experienced a major hormone change?

If you can't think of anything new that has changed, then consider things you have been meaning to change. Do you still use half a dozen chemical products on your skin every day, or continue to use scented candles in every room? As you clean up your body's signals, it will start communicating with you about things it doesn't like. These things may have always been a problem, but because your body couldn't tell you, or it had bigger things to worry about, it was not able to let you know until now. I'll be honest, this looks and feels a lot like your body getting more sensitive. And it is—but not in all the negative ways you may be thinking. It's good for the body to tell us, for example, that the chemicals and poisons that are being put on the skin are harmful. You are choosing to give your body permission to be a speaking partner with you in your health, and it is doing that. Remember, you are both on the same team!

And there is further good news. For most people, once healing is done, those "sensitivities" will be quieter. The body has been created to deal with toxin exposure and, once it is healthy, it will do that well. Lotions, air fresheners, pollution, junk food, and other "toxic" things will not be a problem for your healthy, well-functioning body, if there is limited exposure.

Are You Experiencing a Die-off Reaction?

Do you remember what happens with a die-off reaction (you can review Chapter 6)? Something causes the "bad guys" in the body to die, which releases their stored toxins. This increase in symptoms is called a die-off, or Herxheimer (herx) reaction. This reaction is also a detox reaction. The body deals with these released toxins like it deals with any other toxin in the body. These toxins can cause the same symptoms, and they have to be cleaned up by the body in the same way. However, unlike the toxins already in your body, you have some control over the release of these toxins. As we discussed in chapter 6, anything that kills bad flora will cause a release of these toxins. If you are feeling worse, it may be these toxins that are causing your symptoms. To test this, try stopping or reducing your probiotic intake for a day or two and see if your symptoms decrease. If so, proceed with probiotics and fermented foods more slowly. Take only the dose your body is tolerating, and keep supporting your body to detox! Detox baths and oil pulling can be especially helpful to help your body deal with this reaction. Remember, *die-off symptoms are essentially toxic symptoms, so using the gentle detox methods discussed in this book can be very helpful!*

Are You Experiencing a Healing Reaction?

Sometimes undesirable symptoms are experienced because the immune system is healing. As the immune system becomes stronger, it will react with stronger symptoms. These symptoms could include swelling, pain, itching, skin eruptions, increased allergic reactions, or more frequent illnesses. Although this may feel like you are getting sicker (aka: worse), it's a good sign! It means the immune system is doing what it should! This phenomenon of "increased symptoms occurring *because of* healing" is sometimes called a healing crisis, or healing reaction. As the immune system becomes well-fed and balanced, it gets right to work. If it was severely repressed, the change may be dramatic. Increased or new reactions to foods or other allergens, worsening eczema, hair loss, and joint pain are commonly experienced. If you remember back to chapter 5, these are all symptoms (or by-products) of inflammation, and they mean that your body is addressing issues. Let's look at an example. Think about the symptoms that come with a cold. We can think that a runny nose or a fever should be suppressed, but they are signs that the body is working well! We need mucus to flush out invading microbes, and higher body temperature to aid the body in killing invading germs. These symptoms should not be repressed, they should be allowed—your body is protecting you! Symptoms (signals) from the body may be showing a delayed reaction to a past injury or illness, *or* the response of the body to a current problem. But in either case, they should not be repressed.

Because this healing reaction is not commonly understood, it is important to work with a practitioner who is familiar with how the body looks as it heals. Modern medicine is not familiar with these processes of healing. They equate symptoms with problems, and want to treat (suppress) them instead of figuring out how to support the body in whatever it need.

Find a GAPS Practitioner

Some of you may already be working with a Certified GAPS Practitioner, but many people who do the GAPS protocol do not work with a practitioner. While it is possible to succeed without a practitioner, you are more likely to be successful if you are working with one. If you are reading this chapter because you feel like you are getting worse, or feel like you are missing something (that you can't quite put your finger on) that may be holding you back, it's probably time to find a GAPS practitioner. They are located all over the world, and if you can't find one in your area, many practitioners offer Skype appointments. You can find a list of active GAPS practitioners at www.gaps. me. I also offer some GAPS support, you can find out more details on my website at bewellclinic.net.

If you already work with a GAPS practitioner, pick up the phone and call them! Practitioners can't help you if you don't tell them what's going on. I have observed that one of the keys to successfully healing through this protocol is frequent communication with your GAPS practitioner. And remember, you have an important voice! You are the one who is observing your body every day—share your thoughts on symptoms, connections and patterns. The best success you will get is from working together.

Consider Pausing the Protocol

As we mentioned in the beginning of this book, sometimes the GAPS protocol is not what your body needs right now. During certain metabolic states, if you are causing too much die-off, or during certain seasons of the year, your body may ask for something very different than the GAPS protocol. There are a variety of reasons why GAPS may not be right for your body right now. How do you know if this is what is going on in you? Well, if you feel like you are fighting your body with every food you are eating on GAPS, it may be one of those times. At moments like this, put your best detective hat on and try really listening to your body. Test different foods, or go without them. Try to figure out what it is asking for, even if it is something not in your current stage, or even on the protocol. If it is a persistent desire, then give your body what it is asking for, and observe what happens. If it's the right thing, you will feel better. Gather these observations to discover, with your body as a partner, what the right thing for you to do is *at this time*. Deciding if you should continue the GAPS protocol or not is one of the most challenging things you can encounter while doing the GAPS diet. If this is something you are feel you are facing, please consider talking to a GAPS practitioner to help you figure this out.

With certain diseases like FPIES, and in some other cases, the body is so reactive that it will react to anything—on or off the GAPS diet. In that case, the protocol should be continued, because doing it will help your body heal. If this is you, I do not recommend proceeding until you have established care with a GAPS practitioner.

Stopping the Protocol

For a few people—whose bodies are very malnourished or toxic—continuing the GAPS diet may be dangerous. Some of these people need to do something very different, or need to do something before they can safely do the GAPS protocol. Very few people fall into this category. Most die-off, detox, or sugar withdrawal symptoms, while annoying, are not life threatening. Life threatening symptoms include blue lips and skin from lack of oxygen, high amounts of retained water that affects heart and lung function, unretractable diarrhea that causes severe dehydration, confused mental status (especially if it declined quickly), inability to stay awake during conversation, and a feeling that they are going to die that came on after beginning the GAPS diet. (This feeling is not uncommon in the severely malnourished, and I have worked with several patients who felt this before beginning GAPS. In their cases, that feeling of impending death went away after they started GAPS.)

If any of these serious symptoms occur, quickly give the body what it needs and is asking for, no matter how bad of a "cheat" it seems to be and, in most cases, you should seek medical attention. When the crisis is over, you can try to figure out why it occurred. For example, perhaps it was from a reaction caused by something you ate too much or little of. In this case it may be safe to continue cautiously and under supervision.

For others, the GAPS protocol should be avoided until the reason is known or the person's health is in a different place. Some people feel like this protocol is their only option, but feel unable or unsafe doing it in their homes because of the severity of their condition. There are several facilities around the world that provide around-the-clock medical care, supervision and meals to people having difficulties with reactions, those that need to be isolated from temptation (such as in addictions, anorexia and schizophrenia), or those that simply feel that they do not have the ability or strength to cook. These facilities, run by GAPS Practitioners, are a wonderful option for those that can or need to use them.

Keep Persevering ("Just Keep Swimming . . . ")

We have discussed a few reasons why the GAPS protocol should be stopped, but *most people will benefit from continuing on the GAPS protocol,* despite undesirable symptoms that may occur. The healing process is complicated. Progress does not look like a straight line. There are dips, pauses, detours, sprints, and backtracking. As the body grows stronger, it will deal with things it had put aside. Toxins that were pushed in a dark corner may be swept out, viruses that the body was not quite able to clear may now be dealt with, and signals that were repressed will let their voice be heard. This journey is emotional, but it is worth it—keep pressing forward. Just keep swimming . . .

Additional Support

It has been said before, but it's worth repeating. Healing is a complicated process. Your body has an innate, or built-in, sense that knows what needs healing and how to do it. It needs to communicate with you to let you know what outside input it needs. Sometimes what it needs is not something that you think about, or know about, and help from a natural practitioner is necessary. It's important to build up a support system for yourself, and use it, especially if and when you are unsure what your body is doing. And this may not just be practitioners with a nutrition focus. Acupuncturists, counselors, naturopaths, chiropractors, or many others could be part of the team you need to support you on your journey to better health.

Chapter Nine

What Should You Do Now?

You made it through this book! Great job! Hopefully you have more information and a better understanding of how you can work with your body toward greater healing. But now what? There is no more book to read, and it's time to do something! This can be the most challenging part of any change—when you have gathered the information and it's now time to take action. Well, to ease that transition, here are a few things I suggest you do.

#1 Find a community that supports you. There are a few forums and groups made specifically for the support of people doing GAPS. Find something that works for you! Some GAPS practitioners run a GAPS group locally. You can come join us at Be Well Community (bewellclinic.net). We are a small, but growing community that is supporting each other in our health journeys.

#2 Get a GAPS practitioner. Not everyone needs a GAPS practitioner, but everyone can be helped by one. A list of certified GAPS practitioners can be found at www.gaps.me. There are GAPS providers all over the world, and if you can't find someone in your area, many do Skype appointments as well. Although my primary desire is to educate on a large scale, I also do nutritional consults for individual people. You can find out more, and request an appointment on my website.

#3 Start doing something today. Even if you're not comfortable with committing to the entire GAPS protocol right now, decide on a small way to start, and start! You may start by making and drinking a pot of meat stock every week, or making a simple ferment, or even just getting rid of the oreos in your pantry. It doesn't matter what the step is, or how small it may seem. Decide, and then do it! Then decide something else, and do it! It won't be long before you will be doing more healthy things than you ever thought you could do. If you take no action step after receiving new information, it will only make taking action harder the next time.

#4 Be patient with yourself, and remember that your main goal is always to become an expert detective. Anyone can do what they are told, but there will be more benefit for you if you are the one who understands what is going on in your body. Try to learn from every mistake and trial. When you get in tune with your body, you will have great potential for health. Approach every step on this journey as just that—a worthwhile and essential step, or experience, in this journey of life that adds to who you are as a wonderful, unique person.

#5 Keep trying. No matter what, keep pursuing health. And remember, happiness does not happen when we reach perfect health. Happiness has the potential to happen all the time. Don't get so wrapped up in your journey that you forget others. Help someone else. Listen to someone else's woes without even mentioning yours. Be generous with your time and money. Choose to be grateful, and tell other people that you are! I believe that a major key to the success in my healing journey is my determination to see good in where I was, be thankful for that good, and to sometimes put myself aside and take care of others. Of course, I did not do this perfectly, but it was a habit and choice that I made regularly. To help others do this, I created a daily journal—*My Daily Insights: A GAPS Journal.* Each day has a brief quote and journaling prompt to encourage you to look outwardly in some way. The journal also has a daily checklist for symptoms and space for you to keep track of foods and supplements you should have every day. You can order a copy of the journal on my website www.notesandinsights.com.

I'm excited for you as you use this new information and encouragement to take your next step on this amazing, challenging, and rewarding journey! I wish you all the best. And I would love to hear from you.

Have a wonderful journey. Onward!

Bibliography

Chapter 1

Campbell-McBride, N. (2010). *Gut and Psychology Syndrome*. York, Pennsylvania: Maple Press.

Fallon, S., Enig, M. (2001). *Nourishing Traditions: The Cookbook That Challenges Politically Correct Nutrition and the Diet Dictocrats*. Washington, DC: NewTrends Publishing, Inc.

Grandjean, P., Landrigan, P. (February 14, 2014). Neurobehavioural Effects of Developmental Toxicity. *The Lancet Neurology*, Volume 13, No. 3 p. 330-338. Retrieved from http://www.thelancet.com/journals/laneur/article/PIIS1474-4422(13)70278-3/fulltext

NPR (November 5, 2013). The Invisible Universe of the Human Microbiome. https://www.youtube.com/watch?v=5DTrENdWvvM

Price, W. (2009). *Nutrition and Physical Degeneration*. La Mesa, CA: The Price-Pottenger Nutrition Foundation.

Chapter 2

Campbell-McBride, N. (2010). *Gut and Psychology Syndrome*. York, Pennsylvania: Maple Press.

Chapter 4

Campbell-McBride, N. (August 15, 2014). Feeding Versus Cleansing. http://www.doctor-natasha.com/feeding-versus-cleansing.php

Campbell-McBride, N. (2010). *Gut and Psychology Syndrome*. York, Pennsylvania: Maple Press.

Campbell-McBride, N. (2016). *Put Your Heart in Your Mouth*. York, Pennsylvania: Maple Press.

Conde Nast. (2014). SELFNutritionData. Retrieved November 17, 2016 from http://nutritiondata.self.com/facts/beef-products/3468/2

Conde Nast. (2014). SELFNutritionData. Retrieved November 17, 2016 from http://nutritiondata.self.com/facts/vegetables-and-vegetable-products/2383/2

Fallon, S., Enig, M. (2000). The Skinny on Fats. Retrieved October 19, 2016 from http://www.westonaprice.org/know-your-fats/the-skinny-on-fats/#composition

Masterjohn, C. (December 14, 2004). *Vitamin A: The Forgotten Bodybuilding Nutrient*. Retrieved October 19, 2016 from http://www.westonaprice.org/health-topics/vitamin-a-the-forgotten-bodybuilding-nutrient/

Morell, S., Daniel, K. (2014). *Nourishing Broth: An Old-Fashioned Remedy for the Modern World*. New York: Grand Central Life & Style, pg. 1-46.

Price, W. (2009). *Nutrition and Physical Degeneration*. La Mesa, CA: The Price-Pottenger Nutrition Foundation.

Chapter 5

Campbell-McBride, N. (2010). *Gut and Psychology Syndrome*. York, Pennsylvania: Maple Press. pg 303-305

Encyclopedia Britannica, Inc. (2014). Retrieved November 16, 2016 from http://blogs.britannica.com/2011/02/human-liver-workhorse-body-picture-essay-day/

Issels Integrative Immuno-Oncology. (2015). Retrieved November 16, 2016 from http://issels.com/treatment-summary/importance-of-detoxification/skin/

Masterjohn, C. (November 14, 2015). Saturated Fat Does a Body Good: Exploring the Biological Roles of These Long-Demonized Yet Heroic Nutrients. Professional lecture.

National Institute of Diabetes and Digestive and Kidney Diseases. (May 2014). Retrieved November 16, 2016 from https://www.niddk.nih.gov/health-information/health-topics/Anatomy/kidneys-how-they-work/Pages/anatomy.aspx

Curtis, A., Fagundes, C., Yang, G, et. all. (June 9, 2015). Circadian Control of Innate Immunity in Macrophages by miR-155 Targeting Bmal1. *PNAS*, vol 112 (23). Retrieved from http://www.pnas.org/content/112/23/7231.full

Chapter 6

Campbell-McBride, N. (2010*). Gut and Psychology Syndrome*. York, Pennsylvania: Maple Press.

Explorable.com. Retrieved on November 16, 2016 from https://explorable.com/discovery-of-bacteria

Gevers, D., et. all. (August 14, 2012). The Human Microbiome Project: A Community Resource for the Healthy Human Microbiome. *PLoS Biol* 10(8). Retrieved from http://journals.plos.org/plosbiology/article?id=10.1371/journal.pbio.1001377

Laleva.org (May 14, 2004). Louis Pasteur Vs Antonine Bechamp and The Germ Theory of Disease Causation-1. Retrieved November 16, 2016 from http://www.laleva.org/eng/2004/05/louis_pasteur_vs_antoine_bchamp_and_the_germ_theory_of_disease_causation_1.html

Chapter 7

Campbell-McBride, N. (August 15, 2014). *One Man's Meat is Another Man's Poison!* Retrieved from http://www.doctor-natasha.com/one-mans-meat-another-mans-poison.php.

Chapter 8

Campbell-McBride, N. (2010). *Gut and Psychology Syndrome.* York, Pennsylvania: Maple Press.

Find a GAPS Practitioner. www.gaps.me

Index

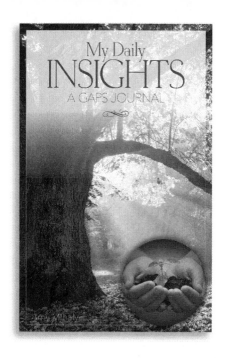

Other Titles by Amy Mihaly

My Daily Insights: A GAPS Journal provides a streamlined approach to track each and every detail that you should monitor while on your health journey. Whether you are healing on your own, or working with a practitioner, this journal is an invaluable tool. On each page you can note your daily symptoms, record your food intake, check off your completed tasks, and take a minute to encourage your heart so you can continue on the journey you have chosen. It is available with a start date of January 1, or with blank dates for a flexible start.

Visit www.notesandinsights.com for more information, or to order.

58036929R00058

Made in the USA
Lexington, KY
01 December 2016